IFFS

STUDIES IN
FERTILITY
AND
STERILITY

Diagnosis and Management of Tubo-Uterine Factors in Infertility

Edited by
R.F. Harrison, J. Bonnar
and W. Thompson

Themes from the XIth World Congress on Fertility and Sterility, Dublin, June 1983, held under the Auspices of the International Federation of Fertility Societies

MTP PRESS LIMITED
a member of the KLUWER ACADEMIC PUBLISHERS GROUP
LANCASTER / BOSTON / THE HAGUE / DORDRECHT

Published in the UK and Europe by
MTP Press Limited
Falcon House
Lancaster, England

British Library Cataloguing in Publication Data

World Congress on Fertility and Sterility
(11th : 1983 : Dublin)
Diagnosis and management of tubo-uterine factors in infertility.—
(Studies in fertility and sterility)
1. Infertility, Female 2. Fallopian tubes 3. Uterus
I. Title II. Harrison, R. F. III. Bonnar, J
IV. Thompson, William, *1937–*
V. International Federation of Fertility Societies
VI. Series 618.1'78 RG201

ISBN-13: 978-94-011-7623-1 e-ISBN-13: 978-94-011-7621-7
DOI: 10.1007/978-94-011-7621-7

Published in the USA by
MTP Press
A division of Kluwer Boston Inc
190 Old Derby Street
Hingham, MA 02043, USA

Library of Congress Cataloging in Publication Data

Main entry under title:
Diagnosis and management of tubo-uterine factors in infertility
(Studies in fertility and sterility)
Includes bibliographical references and index.
1. Infertility–Etiology–Congresses. 2. Fallopian tubes–Diseases–Congresses.
3. Uterus–Diseases–Congresses. I. Harrison, R. F. (Robert Frederick) II. Bonnar, John.
III. Thompson, W. IV. World Congress of Fertility and Sterility (11th : 1983 : Dublin, Dublin) V. International Federation of Fertility Societies. VI. Series.
[DNLM: 1. Fallopian Tube Diseases–congresses. 2. Infertility–etiology–congresses.

Phototypesetting by
Georgia Origination, Liverpool

Butler & Tanner Limited, Frome and London

Contents

CONTENTS

Section 2: Endoscopic Results in Comparison with Other Techniques

PART V: MICROSURGERY

Section 1: Case Selection

Section 2: Special Techniques

Preface

This is the second compilation of papers given during the Related Communications Sessions of the XIth International Federation of Fertility Societies World Congress held on June 26th–July 1st 1983 at the Royal Dublin Society, Dublin, Ireland.

Except for Part I, where results of animal experimentations are gathered together, the volume is concerned solely with studies in the human. The role of infection and endometriosis in the aetiology and treatment of the tubo-uteroperitoneal factor in infertility are the concern of Parts II and III. Diagnostic and therapeutic aspects of tubal disease are covered in Parts IV and V and the book ends with Part VI, chapters on the uterus and vagina.

Laparoscopy and microsurgical techniques have undoubtedly transformed the diagnostic and therapeutic outlook in this area of infertility. This book shows you how far such techniques have progressed and how much there is yet to do.

Dublin, 1983

Robert F. Harrison
John Bonnar
William Thompson

List of Contributors

J. ABE
Department of Obstetrics and Gynecology
Kyoto Prefectural University of Medicine
Kawarmachi-Hirokogi, Kamikyoku, Kyoto
JAPAN 602

M. AL ACHMAR
"Marika Eliadi" Maternity Hospital
2 Helena Venizelos Square
Athens 115 21
GREECE

W. ALBRICH
Department of Obstetrics and Gynecology
University of Munich
Marchioninistrasse
D-8000 Munich 70
WEST GERMANY

J. J. AMY
Department of Obstetrics and Gynecology
Academisch Ziekenhuis - V.U.B.
Larbeeklaan 101
1090 Brussels
BELGIUM

C. ANANDAKUMAR
Department of Obstetrics and Gynaecology
National University of Singapore
Kandang Kerbau Hospital
Hampshire Road
SINGAPORE 0821

A. ARDOIN
Institut Pasteur
Paris
FRANCE

S. A. Z. BADAWY
Department of Obstetrics and Gynecology
Upstate Medical Center
750 E. Adams Street
Syracuse, NY 13210
USA

M. BERG
Department of Clinical Sciences
University of Tampere
Teiskontie 35
SF-33520 Tampere
FINLAND

G. BIRO
University of Saarland
Department of Obstetrics and Gynecology
D-6650 Homburg-Saar
WEST GERMANY

W. D. BOECKX
Centre for Microsurgery
Academic Hospital De Gasthuisberg
University of Leuven
B-3000 Leuven
BELGIUM

M. BOER-MEISEL
Department of Obstetrics and Gynecology
Free University Hospital
de Boelelaan 1117
1007 NB Amsterdam
THE NETHERLANDS

A. BÖGER
Zentrum für Pathologie
Philipps-Universität Marburg
Robert-Koch-Strasse 5
D-3550 Marburg
WEST GERMANY

P. R. BOWMAN
Coombe Lying-in Hospital
Cork Street
Dublin 8
IRELAND

I. BROSENS
Department of Obstetrics and Gynecology
University Hospital St. Rafaël-Gasthuisberg
Herestraat, 49
B-3000 Leuven
BELGIUM

P. BUSSIERE
Hôpital Jean Rostand
92310 Sèvres
FRANCE

H. M. BUVAT
Association Etude de la Pathologie de L'Appareil Reproducteur
49 Rue de la Bassée
59000 Lille
FRANCE

J. BUVAT
Association Etude de la Pathologie de L'Appareil Reproducteur
49 Rue de la Bassée
59000 Lille
FRANCE

S. CAMPO
Department of Obstetrics and Gynecology
Universita' Cattolica Sacro Cuore
Largo A. Gemelli
00168 Roma
ITALY

F. CATALAN
Institut Fournier
Paris
FRANCE

R. CEVENINI
Institute of Microbiology
University of Bologna
Bologna
ITALY

C. CIGARINI
Department of Obstetrics and Gynaecology
Santa Maria Nuova Hospital
42100 Reggio Emilia
ITALY

R. CITTADINO
Department of Obstetrics and Gynecology
Upstate Medical Center
750 E. Adams Street
Syracuse, NY 13210
USA

A. C. COMNINOS
"Marika Eliadi" Maternity Hospital
20 Kanari Street
Athens 106 73
GREECE

V. CUENCA
Department of Obstetrics and Gynecology
Upstate Medical Center
750 E. Adams Street
Syracuse, NY 13210
USA

C. CUVELIER
Association Etude de la Pathologie de L'Appareil Reproducteur
49 Rue de la Bassée
59000 Lille
FRANCE

M. DARLING
Rotunda Hospital
Dublin 1
IRELAND

J. DE BRUX
Institut de Pathologie et Cytologie Appliquée
B.P. 450-16-75769 Paris Cédex 16
FRANCE

F. DESMONS
Association Etude de la Pathologie de L'Appareil Reproducteur
49 Rue de la Bassée
59000 Lille
FRANCE

LIST OF CONTRIBUTORS

L. DESSANTI
Department of Obstetrics and Gynaecology
Santa Maria Nuova Hospital
42100 Reggio Emilia
ITALY

D. DEVRIES
Department of Obstetrics and Gynaecology
Haifa Medical Center (Rothschild)
Faculty of Medicine - Technion
47 Golomb Street, PO Box 4940
Haifa 321048
ISRAEL

C. DINCER
Universitäts-Klinikum Charlottenburg
Pulsstrasse 4
D-1000 Berlin 19
WEST GERMANY

P. J. DÖRR
Department of Obstetrics and Gynecology
Westeinde Hospital
Lijnbaan 32
2501 CH Den Haag
THE NETHERLANDS

N. M. DUIGNAN
Coombe Lying-in Hospital
Cork Street
Dublin 8
IRELAND

F. P. EHRLING-SIMKE
University of Saarland
Department of Obstetrics and Gynecology
D-6650 Homburg-Saar
WEST GERMANY

I. EIBSCHITZ
Department of Obstetrics and Gynaecology
Haifa Medical Center (Rothschild)
Faculty of Medicine - Technion
47 Golomb Street, P.O. Box 4940
Haifa 31048
ISRAEL

G. ENAULT
28 rue Ponthieu
75-008 Paris
FRANCE

M. ERDREICH
Psychiatric Services
Haifa Medical Center (Rothschild)
Faculty of Medicine - Technion
47 Golomb Street, P.O. Box 4940
Haifa 31048
ISRAEL

J. L. H. EVERS
Department of Obstetrics and Gynaecology
St. Annadal Academic Hospital
University of Limburg
P.O. Box 1918
6201 BX Maastricht
THE NETHERLANDS

M. S. FOSCOLU
Department of Obstetrics and Gynaecology
Franchini Hospital
42027 Montecchio (Reggio Emilia)
ITALY

W. FOULON
Department of Obstetrics and Gynecology
Academisch Ziekenhuis - V.U.B.
Laarbeeklaan, 101
1090 Brussels
BELGIUM

J. C. FOURLINNIE
Association Etude de la Pathologie de
L'Appareil Reproducteur
49 rue de la Bassée
59000 Lille
FRANCE

T. FUJIWARA
Department of Obstetrics and Gynecology
School of Medicine, Keio University
35 Shinanomachi, Shinjuku-ku Tokyo 160
JAPAN

N. GARCEA
Department of Obstetrics and Gynecology
Universita' Cattolica Santa Cuore
Largo A. Gemelli
00168 Roma
ITALY

G. GHIRARDINI
Department of Obstetrics and Gynaecology
Franchini Hospital
42027 Montecchio (Reggio Emilia)
ITALY

E. GIACCHI
Department of Obstetrics and Gynecology
Universita' Cattolica Sacro Cuore
Largo A. Gemelli
00168 Roma
ITALY

S. GORDTS
Department of Obstetrics and Gynecology
University Hospital St. Rafaël-Gasthuisberg
Herestraat, 49
B-3000 Leuven
BELGIUM

A. GÖTZ
Department of Obstetrics and Gynecology
University of Munich
Marchioninistrasse
D-8000 Munich 70
WEST GERMANY

M. GRANAT
Department of Obstetrics and Gynecology
Hadassah University Hospital
Ein Kerem, PO Box 12000
Jerusalem
ISRAEL

A. T. GREENE
Coombe Lying-in Hospital
Cork Street
Dublin 8
IRELAND

W. GRUENBERGER
1st Department of Gynecology and Obstetrics
Vienna University - Spitalgasse 23
A-1090 Vienna
AUSTRIA

D. SOJO GUTTERO
Fertility Unit
Centro Especial "Ramón y Cajal"
Crta. de Colmenar Km. 9,100
Madrid 34
SPAIN

C. HAMMER
Institute for Surgical Research Grosshadern
University of Munich
Marchioninistrasse
D-8000 Munich 70
WEST GERMANY

A. G. J. M. HANSELAAR
Department of Pathology
St. Radboud University Hospital
Geert Grooteplein Zuid 24
6525 GA Nijmegen
THE NETHERLANDS

R. HARRISON
Rotunda Hospital
Dublin 1
IRELAND

R. HARTWIG
Universitäts-Klinikum Charlottenburg
Pulsstrasse 4
D-1000 Berlin 19
WEST GERMANY

T. HASHIMOTO
Department of Obstetrics and Gynecology
School of Medicine, Keio University
35 Shinanomachi Shinjuku-ku Tokyo 160
JAPAN

P. K. HEINONEN
Department of Obstetrics and Gynecology
University Central Hospital
Teiskontie 35
SF-33520 Tampere
FINLAND

J. HENRY-SUCHET
Hôpital Jean Rostand
141 Grand rue
92310 Sèvres
FRANCE

H. HEPP
University of Saarland
Department of Obstetrics and Gynecology
D-6650 Homburg-Saar
WEST GERMANY

J. C. HERBAUT
Association Etude de la Pathologie de L'Appareil Reproducteur
49 rue de la Bassée
59000 Lille
FRANCE

C. J. HERMAN
Department of Pathology
St. Radboud University Hospital
Geert Grooteplein Zuid 24
6525 GA Nijmegen
THE NETHERLANDS

LIST OF CONTRIBUTORS

G. HOLCBERG
Division of Obstetrics and Gynecology
Soroka Medical Center
Beer Sheva 84120
ISRAEL

H. W. HORNE
Department of Obstetrics and Gynecology
Harvard Medical School
1330 Boylston Street, Chestnut Hill
MA 02167
USA

H. HOSHIAI
Department of Obstetrics and Gynecology
Tohoku University School of Medicine
1-1 Seiryo-machi, Sendai 980
JAPAN

R. IIZUKA
Department of Obstetrics and Gynecology
School of Medicine, Keio University
35 Shinanomachi, Shinjuku-ku Tokyo 160
JAPAN

H. IMAIZUMI
Department of Obstetrics and Gynecology
Tohoku University School of Medicine
1-1 Seiryo-machi, Sendai 980
JAPAN

V. INSLER
Division of Obstetrics and Gynecology
Soroka Medical Center
Beer Sheva 84120
ISRAEL

R. D. B. JACOBS
Department of Obstetrics and Gynecology
Upstate Medical Center
750 E. Adams Street
Syracuse, NY 13210
USA

M. J. JAMES
Department of Surgery
Flinders Medical Centre
Bedford Park
SOUTH AUSTRALIA 5042

H. JANISCH
2nd Department of Obstetrics and Gynaecology
Spitalgasse 23
A-1090 Vienna
AUSTRIA

R. S. JEYENDRAN
Institute of Reproductive Medicine
III N. Wabash Avenue, Suite 106
Chicago, IL 60602
USA

W. R. JONES
Department of Obstetrics and Gynaecology
Flinders Medical Centre
Bedford Park
SOUTH AUSTRALIA 5042

Y. KANEKO
Department of Obstetrics and Gynecology
Toho University Hospital
6-11-1 Ohmori Nishi, Ota-ku, Tokyo
JAPAN 143

I. KAPLAN
Department of Plastic Surgery
Beilinson Medical Center
Petah Tiqva 49 100
ISRAEL

Z. KATZ
Department of Obstetrics and Gynecology
Kaplan Hospital
76-100 Rehovot
ISRAEL

A. KAUPPILA
Department of Obstetrics and Gynecology
University of Oulu
SF-90220 Oulu
FINLAND

J. KAVVOS
1st Obstetrical and Gynaecological Clinic
"Marika Eliadi" Maternity Hospital
1 Semitelou Street
GR-11528 Athens
GREECE

S. KAWAKAMI
Department of Obstetrics and Gynecology
School of Medicine, Keio University
35 Shinanomachi, Shinjuku-ku, Tokyo 160
JAPAN

N. KIMMEL
Virology Unit
Soroka University Hospital and Faculty of Health Sciences
Beer Sheva 84120
ISRAEL

J. KIMURA
Department of Obstetrics and Gynecology
Kyoto Prefectural University of Medicine
Kawaramachi-Hirokogi, Kamikyoku, Kyoto
JAPAN

D. KLEINMAN
Division of Obstetrics and Gynecology
Soroka University Hospital and Faculty of Health Sciences
Ben Gurion University of the Negev
Beer Sheva 84120
ISRAEL

E. KOJIMA
Department of Obstetrics and Gynecology
Toho University Hospital
6-11-1 Ohmori Nishi, Ota-ku, Tokyo
JAPAN

Ch. KRÜGER
Bundesgesundheitsamt, Max von Pettenkover-Institut, Unter den Eichen 82
D-1000 Berlin 45
WEST GERMANY

E. KUBISTA
1st Department of Gynecology and Obstetrics
Vienna University, Spitalgasse 23
A-1090 Vienna
AUSTRIA

R.B. KUNDSIN
Department of Microbiology
Harvard Medical School
Brigham and Women's Hospital
75 Francis Street
Boston, MA 02115
USA

G.C. LA SALA
Department of Obstetrics and Gynaecology
Santa Maria Nuova Hospital
42100 Reggio Emilia
ITALY

M. LAHTINEN
Department of Clinical Sciences
University of Tampere
Teiskontie 35
SF-33520 Tampere
FINLAND

T. LAINAS
"Marika Eliadi" Maternity Hospital
2 Helena Venizelos Square
Athens 115 21
GREECE

M. LANCET
Department of Obstetrics and Gynecology
Kaplan Hospital
76-100 Rehovot
ISRAEL

J.A. LAND
Department of Obstetrics and Gynaecology
St. Annadal Academic Hospital
University of Limburg, PO Box 1918
6201 BX Maastricht
THE NETHERLANDS

M. LANGER
1st Department of Gynecology and Obstetrics
Vienna University, Spitalgasse 23
A-1090 Vienna
AUSTRIA

A. LEADER
Endocrine/Infertility Clinic
University of Calgary Medical Clinic
3330-Hospital Drive N.W.
Calgary, Alberta T2N 4N1
CANADA

A. LEMAIRE
Association Etude de la Pathologie de L'Appareil Reproducteur
49 rue de la Bassée
59000 Lille
FRANCE

V. LOFFREDO
Hôpital Jean Rostand
141 Grand rue
92310 Sèvres
FRANCE

T. LOYSEL
Hôpital Jean Rostand
141 Grand rue
92310 Sèvres
FRANCE

J. E. LÜTTGES
Zentrum für Pathologie
Philipps-Universität Marburg
Robert-Koch-Strasse 5
D-3550 Marburg
WEST GERMANY

V. MAASSEN
Department of Gynecology and Obstetrics
Berlin - Charlottenburg
Free University Berlin
Pulstrasse 4
D-1000 Berlin 19
WEST GERMANY

S. MAKABE
Department of Obstetrics and Gynecology
Toho University Hospital
6-11-1 Ohmori Nishi, Ota Ku, Tokyo
JAPAN

E. J. MARGALIOTH
Department of Obstetrics and Gynecology
Hadassah University Hospital
91 120 Jerusalem
ISRAEL

L. MARSHALL
Department of Obstetrics and Gynecology
Upstate Medical Center
750 E. Adams Street
Syracuse, NY 13210
USA

K. MAVRELOS
Maternity Hospital "Marika Eliadi"
Athens
GREECE

P. J. MCKENNA
Rotunda Hospital
Dublin 1
IRELAND

A. MESHORER
Animal Experimental Department
Weizmann Institute of Science
76-100 Rehovot
ISRAEL

M. MESSINA
Department of Obstetrics and Gynecology
Universita' Cattolica Sacro Cuore
Largo A. Gemelli
00168 Roma
ITALY

M. METKA
1st Department of Gynecology and Obstetrics
Vienna University, Spitalgasse 23
Vienna
AUSTRIA

M. MINTZ
211 rue de l'Université
75007 Paris
FRANCE

K. MIYAZAKI
Department of Obstetrics and Gynecology
Osaka Medical College
2-7 Daigakucho, Takasuki, Osaka 569
JAPAN

K. MOMOSE
Department of Obstetrics and Gynecology
Toho University Hospital
6-11-1 Ohmon Nishi, Ota-ku, Tokyo
JAPAN 143

S. MOR-YOSEF
Department of Obstetrics and Gynecology
Hadassah University Hospital
91 120 Jerusalem
ISRAEL

R. MORI
Department of Obstetrics and Gynecology
Tohoku University School of Medicine
1-1 Seiryo-machi, Sendai 980
JAPAN

M. MORISADA
Department of Obstetrics and Gynecology
School of Medicine, Keio University
35 Shinanomachi, Shinjuku-ku, Tokyo 160
JAPAN

T. J. MUDGE
Department of Obstetrics and Gynaecology
Flinders Medical Centre
Bedford Park
SOUTH AUSTRALIA 5042

A. NAESSENS
Department of Microbiology
Academisch Ziekenhuis - V.U.B.
Laarbeeklaan, 101
1090 Brussels
BELGIUM

D. NAVOT
Department of Obstetrics and Gynecology
Hadassah University Hospital
91 120 Jerusalem
ISRAEL

S. NITSCHKE-DABELSTEIN
Universitäts-Frauenklinik Marburg
Philipps-Universität Marburg
Pilgrimstein 3
D-3550 Marburg
WEST GERMANY

M. NUSBAUM
Department of Obstetrics and Gynecology
Upstate Medical Center
750 E. Adams Street
Syracuse, NY 13210
USA

H. OKADA
Department of Obstetrics and Gynecology
Kyoto Prefectural University of Medicine
Kawaramachi-Hirokogi, Kamikyoku, Kyoto
JAPAN 602

G. OMURA
Department of Obstetrics and Gynecology
Toho University Hospital
6-11-1 Ohmori Nishi, Ota-ku, Tokyo
JAPAN 143

B.C. OOI
Institute of Health
Outram Road
SINGAPORE 0316

J. OVADIA
Department of Obstetrics and Gynecology
Beilinson Medical Center
Petah Tiqva 49 100
ISRAEL

J. PAAVONEN
Department of Clinical Sciences
University of Tampere
Teiskontie 35
SF-33520 Tampere
FINLAND

R. PALMER
87 Boulevard Berthier
75-017 Paris
FRANCE

V. PANETTA
Department of Obstetrics and Gynecology
Universita' Cattolica Sacro Cuore
Largo A. Gemelli
00168 Roma
ITALY

F.X. PARIS
Hôpital Jean Rostand 92310
Sèvres
FRANCE

H.A. PATTINSON
Endocrine/Infertility Clinic
University of Calgary Medical Clinic
3330-Hospital Drive N.W.
Calgary, Alberta T2N 4N1
CANADA

M. PEREZ-PELAEZ
Institute of Reproductive Medicine
111 N. Wabash Avenue, Suite 1016
Chicago, IL 60602
USA

C. PETERS-WELTE
Department of Obstetrics and Gynecology
Grosshadern University of Munich
Marchioninistrasse
D-8000 Munich 70
WEST GERMANY

J.P. PEZ
Hôpital Jean Rostand 92310
Sèvres
FRANCE

R. PIJNENBORG
Unit for the Study of Human Reproduction
Academic Hospital De Gasthuisberg
University of Leuven
B-3000 Leuven
BELGIUM

G. POEHNER
Department of Gynecology and Obstetrics
Berlin - Charlottenburg
Free University Berlin
Pulsstrasse 4
D-1000 Berlin 19
WEST GERMANY

G. POTASHNIK
Division of Obstetrics and Gynecology
Soroka Medical Center
Beer Sheva 84120
ISRAEL

LIST OF CONTRIBUTORS

J. CORTÉS PRIETO
Fertility Unit
Centro Especial "Ramón y Cajal"
Crta. de Colmenar Km. 9,100
Madrid 34
SPAIN

U. PUDLO
Department of Gynecology and Obstetrics
Pilgrimstein 2
355 Marburg
WEST GERMANY

E. RADKE
Universitäts-Klinikum Charlottenburg
Pulsstrasse 4
D-1000 Berlin 19
WEST GERMANY

H. RAJANIEMI
Department of Anatomy
University of Oulu
SF-90220 Oulu 22
FINLAND

S. S. RATNAM
Department of Obstetrics and Gynaecology
National Kerbau Hospital
Hampshire Road
SINGAPORE 0821

M. RAUFF
Department of Obstetrics and Gynaecology
National University of Singapore
Kandang Kerbau Hospital
Hampshire Road
SINGAPORE 0821

P. RISS
2nd Department of Obstetrics and Gynaecology
Spitalgasse 23
A-1090 Vienna
AUSTRIA

Y. ROBERT
Hôpital Jean Rostand
141 Grand rue
92310 Sèvres
FRANCE

A. M. ROGAN
Department of Obstetrics and Gynaecology
University Hospital, Anichstrasse 35
A-6020 Innsbruck
AUSTRIA

L. RÖNNBERG
Department of Obstetrics and Gynecology
University of Oulu
SF-90220 Oulu
FINLAND

D. ROZENMAN
Department of Obstetrics and Gynecology
Kaplan Hospital
76-100 Rehovot
ISRAEL

P. CUEVAS SÁNCHEZ
Research Department (Histology)
Centro Especial "Ramón y Cajal"
Crta. de Colmenar Km. 9,100
Madrid 34
SPAIN

B. SAROV
Epidemiology Unit, Faculty of Health Sciences
Ben Gurion University of the Negev
Beer Sheva 84120
ISRAEL

I. SAROV
Virology Unit, Faculty of Health Sciences
Ben Gurion University of the Negev
Beer Sheva 84120
ISRAEL

S. SARRIS
Maternity Hospital "Marika Eliadi"
26 Timoleondos Vassou
Athens 115-21
GREECE

P. SCHEIDEL
University of Saarland
Department of Obstetrics and Gynecology
D-6650 Hamburg-Saar
WEST GERMANY

J. G. SCHENKER
Department of Obstetrics and Gynecology
Hadassah University Hospital
91 120 Jerusalem
ISRAEL

K. SCHIEDER
2nd Department of Obstetrics and Gynaecology
Spitalgasse 23
A-1090 Vienna
AUSTRIA

D. SCHMIDT
3 rue des Cottages
75 018 Paris
FRANCE

M. SCHWERDT
Universitäts-Klinikum Charlottenburg
Pulsstrasse 4
D-1000 Berlin 19
WEST GERMANY

E. SEDBON
32 rue de la Colonie
75 013 Paris
FRANCE

D. SERFATY
Centre de Fertilité
Hôpital Saint Louis
Paris
FRANCE

M. SHARF
Department of Obstetrics and Gynaecology
Haifa Medical Center (Rothschild)
Faculty of Medicine-Technion
47 Golomb Street, PO Box 4940
Haifa 31048
ISRAEL

H. SHIHOR
Psychiatric Services
Haifa Medical Center (Rothschild)
Faculty of Medicine-Technion
47 Golomb Street, PO Box 4940
Haifa 31048
ISRAEL

A. J. SOBRERO
Institute of Reproductive Medicine
111 N. Wabash Avenue, Suite 1016
Chicago, IL 60602
USA

A. SOLER
Hôpital Jean Rostand
141 Grand rue
92310 Sèvres
FRANCE

H. SPIELMANN
Bundesgesundheitsamt, Max von Pettenkover-Institut, Unter den Eichen 82
D-1000 Berlin 45
WEST GERMANY

Ch. STADLER
Department of Gynecology and Obstetrics
Berlin-Charlottenburg
Free University Berlin, Pulsstrasse 4
D-1000 Berlin 19
WEST GERMANY

M. STAUBER
Universitäts-Klinikum Charlottenburg
Pulsstrasse 4
D-1000 Berlin 19
WEST GERMANY

A. STITZEL
Pediatrics Department
Upstate Medical Center
750 E. Adams Street
Syracuse, NY 13210
USA

O. SUGIMOTO
Department of Obstetrics and Gynecology
Osaka Medical College
2-7 Daigakucho, Takasuki, Osaka 569
JAPAN

M. SUZUKI
Department of Obstetrics and Gynecology
Tohoku University School of Medicine
1-1 Seiryo-machi, Sendai 980
JAPAN

Y. TADIR
Department of Obstetrics and Gynecology
Beilinson Medical Center
Petah Tiqva 49 100
ISRAEL

K. TAKAHASHI
Department of Obstetrics and Gynecology
Sendai National Hospital
2-8-8 Miyagino, Sendai 983
JAPAN

T. TAMAYA
Department of Obstetrics and Gynecology
Kyoto Prefectural University of Medicine
Kawaramachi-Hirokogi, Kamikyoku, Kyoto
JAPAN 602

P. J. TAYLOR
Endocrine/Infertility Clinic
University of Calgary Medical Clinic
3330 Hospital Drive N.W.
Calgary, Alberta T2N 4N1
CANADA

L. TESQUIER
Hôpital Jean Rostand
141 Grand rue
92310 Sèvres
FRANCE

R.H. TOMAR
Clinic Pathology
Upstate Medical Center
750 E. Adams Street
Syracuse, NY 13210
USA

J. TORT GRUMBACH
Hôpital Jean Rostand
92310 Sèvres
FRANCE

E. TSAMANIS
"Marika Eliadi" Maternity Hospital
2 Helena Venizelos Square
Athens 115 21
GREECE

S. UEHARA
Department of Obstetrics and Gynecology
Tohoku University School of Medicine
1-1 Seiryo-machi, Sendai 980
JAPAN

F. VALLI
Department of Obstetrics and Gynaecology
Santa Maria Nuova Hospital
421000 Reggio Emilia
ITALY

H.M. VEMER
Department of Obstetrics and Gynecology
St. Radboud University Hospital
Geert Grooteplein Zuid 1
6525 GA Nijmegen
THE NETHERLANDS

M. VOLCKAERT
Department of Obstetrics and Gynecology
Academisch Ziekenhuis - V.U.B.
Laarbeeklaan, 101
1090 Brussels
BELGIUM

J. A. WALSH
Department of Surgery, Flinders Medical Centre
Bedford Park
SOUTH AUSTRALIA 5042

R. WIEDEMANN
University of Saarland
Department of Obstetrics and Gynecology
D-6650 Homburg-Saar
WEST GERMANY

P.C. WONG
Department of Obstetrics and Gynaecology
National University of Singapore
Kandang Kerbau Hospital
Hampshire Road
SINGAPORE 0821

M. YEMINI
Department of Obstetrics and Gynecology
Kaplan Hospital
76-100 Rehovot
ISRAEL

Z. ZUCKERMAN
Department of Obstetrics and Gynecology
Beilinson Medical Center
Petah Tiqva 49 100
ISRAEL

G. ZWIENS
Universitäts-Frauenklinik Marburg
Philipps-Universität Marburg
Pilgrimstein 3
D-3550 Marburg
WEST GERMANY

E. ZYLBER-KATZ
Medicine A, Clinical Pharmacology Unit
Hadassah University Hospital
EinKerem, PO Box 12000
Jerusalem
ISRAEL

Part I

The Animal Oviduct

Part I

Section 1: Physiology

1
The impact of tubal surgery on early embryonic development in the rabbit oviduct

J. L. H. EVERS, J. A. LAND, R. PIJNENBORG, W. D. BOECKX and I. A. BROSENS

INTRODUCTION

The effect of tubal surgery upon reproductive processes in the oviduct is still incompletely understood. Results of surgery usually are expressed by means of a postoperative tubal patency test or by measuring the nidation index[1].

Halbert *et al.*[2], Perez *et al.*[3] and McComb *et al.*[4] studied the transport function of the oviduct following surgery. The present study was undertaken to examine the effect of tubal surgery upon early embryonic development in the rabbit oviduct.

MATERIALS AND METHODS

Twenty-one virgin rabbits of the Dutch belted strain were used in these experiments. In 11 rabbits a resection–reanastomosis of one oviduct was performed with microsurgical techniques as reported earlier[1]. The contralateral non-operated oviduct served as a first-order control. The remaining 10 animals were not operated on and served as a second-order control. After 3–13 weeks postoperatively each doe was mated with a buck of proven fertility after 125 IU human chorionic gonadotrophin were given to ensure ovulation.

23–25 hours after mating the doe was killed, both oviducts excised and flushed with Earl's solution. The flushings were checked for embryos and their cleavage stage was recorded. Except for the surgery the same procedure was applied to the control animals.

RESULTS

All of the surgically altered oviducts appeared to be patent when flushing was performed.

One hundred and thirteen corpora lutea were counted in the 21 rabbits. Ninety-three ova could be retrieved, representing an ovum recovery rate of 82.3%. Fifteen ova were found to be degenerating: three in the control animals and 12 in the experimental group. The 12 ova in the experimental group concerned four ova in the control tubes and eight in the operated tubes. The distribution of the remaining 78 embryos according to developmental stage is shown in Table 1.

Table 1 Distribution of 78 embryos according to developmental stage in the tubes of 11 non-operated control animals (CA), in the contralateral control tubes of the 10 operated animals (CT) and in the operated tubes of the operated animals (OT)

	Developmental stage			
Group	*1-cell*	*2-cell*	*4-cell*	*8-cell*
CA	29 (69%)	12 (29%)	1 (2%)	0 (0%)
CT	6 (30%)	8 (40%)	5 (25%)	1 (5%)
OT	3 (19%)	10 (63%)	3 (19%)	0 (0%)

The χ^2 determination of difference between the developmental stages of embryos in the control animals, control tubes and operated tubes indicated a significant difference between the cleavage stages of embryos in the control animals and control tubes ($p<0.01$), and between the embryos in the control animals and operated tubes ($p<0.001$). The differences between the develop-

Table 2 Distribution of the 36 embryos in the control tubes and in the operated tubes of the operated animals according to developmental stage and surgery-mating interval duration

Developmental stage	*No. of embryos*										
1-cell	2	–	–	–	–	2	1	–	–	–	4
2-cell	11	2	–	–	–	–	3	–	2	–	–
4-cell	6	2	–	–	–	–	–	–	–	–	–
8-cell	1	–	–	–	–	–	–	–	–	–	–
Interval (weeks)	03	04	05	06	07	08	09	10	11	12	13

mental stages in the control tubes and operated tubes appeared not to be significant.

As shown in Table 2 a tendency existed for the higher cleavage rates to occur in rabbits which had been mated in the first few weeks of their postoperative recovery period.

DISCUSSION

In rabbits copulation is followed by ovulation in 10–12 hours[5]. No exact figures are known concerning the cleavage rate of rabbit embryos during tubal transport. The present investigation showed 69% of the embryos in the control animals to be in the one-cell stage 23–25 hours after mating (Table 1). Almost all of the remainder were two-cell embryos (29%). After the same interval in the operated animals 63% of the embryos in the operated tube, and 40% of the embryos in the non-operated control tubes, had progressed to the two-cell stage. 4 and 8-cell cleavage stages were found in 19% of the embryos in the operated tubes and in 30% of the embryos in the control tubes.

The results of our study suggest an embryonic cleavage promoting factor to be more active in the operated animals. This factor seems to affect not only the operated tube but the contralateral tube as well. The action of this factor appears to be more pronounced the sooner the animals were mated after the operation. Urzua *et al.*[6] described a macromolecular protein (blastokinin or uteroglobin) to be present in uterine fluid of pregnant rabbits. The appearance of this protein (molecular weight, 28 000) was provoked by progesterone. Blastokinin was shown to affect the *in vitro* development of preimplantation embryos. Roblero and Izquierdo[7] demonstrated the presence of a special macromolecular protein fraction in mouse serum. This protein bound to progesterone and stimulated the cleavage rate of early embryos. They found a significant increase in the mean number of blastomeres per blastocyst when embryos were cultured in a medium supplemented with this macromolecular fraction of serum in the presence of progesterone. There was no progesterone effect in the absence of this macromolecular serum fraction.

Blastokinin is thought to be able to bind progesterone and to stimulate the growth of rabbit blastocysts and the uptake of nucleosides and amino acids. Stone *et al.*[8] found significantly fewer pronuclear rabbit zygotes developing normally to the morula stage in oestrogen-influenced oviduct fluid, compared with zygotes in progesterone influenced fluid. They suggested the existence of an oestrogen mediated, low molecular weight (<10 000 daltons) inhibitor of embryonic development to be present in oviduct fluid.

In our group of animals the rate of early embryonic development was stimulated following tubal surgery. This can be due to an increase of blastokinin or an alike growth promoting factor, or to a decrease of a growth inhibitor.

Postoperative enhancement of embryonic development in the human could be an additional reason for the increased rate of occurrence of ectopic pregnancies following tubal surgery, even in the non-operated oviduct. The fact that the first pregnancy following infertility microsurgery often ends in an abortion might also be explained by the changes in early embryonic development following tubal surgery.

References

1. Boeckx, W. D. (1983). *Reconstructive Microsurgery of the Rabbit Oviduct*. Academic Thesis, Leuven
2. Halbert, S. A., McComb, P. F. and Bourdage, R. J. (1981). The structural and functional impact of microsurgical anastomosis on the rabbit oviductal isthmus. *Fertil. Steril.*, **36**, 653
3. Perez, I. D., Rajkumar, K. and Eddy, C. A. (1981). Fertility and ovum transport after microsurgical removal of the uterotubal junction in rabbits. *Fertil. Steril.*, **36**, 803
4. McComb, P. F., Newman, H. and Halbert, S. A. (1981). Reproduction in rabbits after excision of the oviductal isthmus, ampullary-isthmic junction and uteroisthmic junction. *Fertil. Steril.*, **36**, 669
5. Younglai, E. V. (1972). Effect of mating on follicular fluid steroids in the rabbit. *J. Reprod. Fertil.*, **30**, 157
6. Urzua, M. A., Stambaugh, R., Flickinger, G. and Mastroianni, L. (1970). Uterine and oviduct fluid protein patterns in the rabbit before and after ovulation. *Fertil. Steril.*, **21**, 860
7. Roblero, L. and Izquierdo, L. (1976). Effect of progesterone on the cleavage rate of mouse embryos *in vitro*. *J. Reprod. Fertil.*, **46**, 475
8. Stone, S. L., Richardson, L. L., Hamner, C. E. and Oliphant, G. (1977). Partial characterization of hormone-mediated inhibition of embryo development in rabbit oviduct fluid. *Biol. Reprod.*, **16**, 647

2
Transport of proteins and water out of an artificial hydrosalpinx in the rabbit

R. WIEDEMANN, P. SCHEIDEL, F. P. EHRLING-SIMKE, G. BIRO and H. HEPP

The hydrosalpinx and the inflammatory reaction that accompanies it are a major problem in the surgical correction of distal tubal occlusion. The inflammatory reaction in chronic salpingitis leads to the formation of fibrotic tissue in the fallopian tube.

In our opinion, the physical transformations induced by the hydrosalpinx, such as flattening of the epithelium and the distension of the tubal lumen, are reversible. In this study, we attempted to demonstrate that a hydrosalpinx without an inflammatory reaction does not damage a tube irreversibly and thus will not require a surgical correction without desire for children. It must be pointed out that observations from this or any other experimental animal study are not necessarily transferable to other animals or even humans. This is particularly important because an acute pelvic inflammatory disease similar to that found in humans has not yet been successfully generated in experimental animals.

From our experience in 48 induced hydrosalpinx we can summarize the effects of the hydrosalpinx in rabbits as:

(1) Distension of the tube independent of the duration of the ligature, i.e. generally volume constancy.
   (a) Flattening of the longitudinal endosalpinx folds.
   (b) Decrease of the epithelium height (cubic).
   (c) Reduction of the strength of the tunica muscularis.

(2) No irreversible morphological changes.
 (a) Increased protrusion due to the hydrosalpinx.

Figure 1 shows a representative section of a hydrosalpinx. Particular attention should be given to the prominent secretory cells in the pre-protrusion stage. The observation made over a period of 6 months demonstrated a volume constancy in the hydrosalpinx which promoted us to take a closer look at the responsible exchange mechanisms. From the electron-microscopic findings we concluded that a paracellular transport may exist. The dispersed intercellular spaces are particularly conspicuous in this figure. A water exchange similar to that found in the intestines seems plausible.

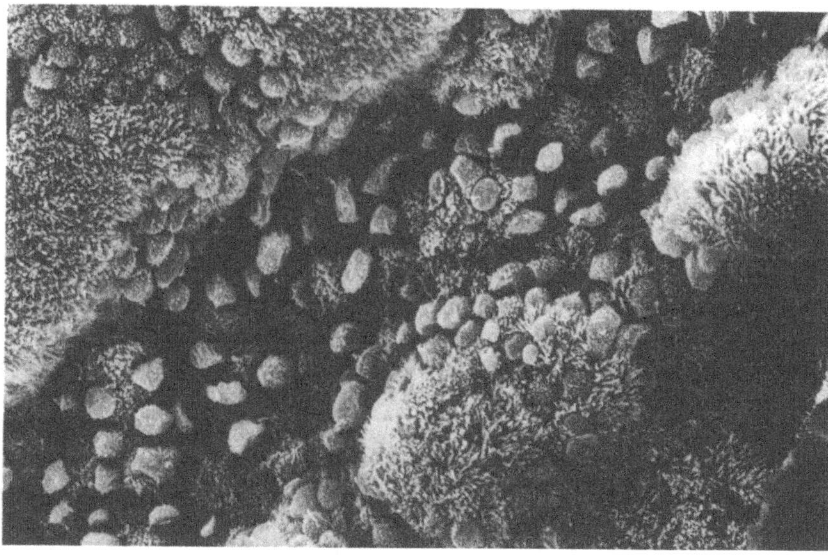

Figure 1 Scanning electron micrograph of the ampullar part of 8-week hydrosalpinx

We attempted to determine the reabsorption of water and proteins out of the tubal lumen with radioactively labelled substances.

PROCEDURE

A mixed breed of adult female rabbits each weighing approximately 3.5 kg were used in this experiment. One tube in each animal was tied off distally and proximally with 3.0 nylon suture material. All animals were administered 75 IU hCG (Prolan R) for synchronization 10 days postoperatively. The relaparotomy was conducted 5 days after hCG administration. All animals demonstrated a well-developed hydrosalpinx. We injected 0.25 ml radioactively labelled substances into the hydrosalpinx of each animal (Table 1). We than measured the serum concentrations of these substances after 5 minutes until 2 weeks after injection.

Table 1 Site, and number of rabbits receiving radiolabels

No. of rabbits	*Substance*	*Injection site*
5	Tritium	Fallopian tube
3	[^{125}I]Albumin	Fallopian tube
3	[^{125}I]hGH	Fallopian tube
2	Tritium	Peritoneum
2	[^{125}I]hGH	Peritoneum

The animals were killed after the last measurements and the remaining activity was measured in the tube. Two animals served as controls. They were given the same initial concentration of radioactively labelled substances to determine the reabsorption across the peritoneum.

Figure 2 shows the serum concentrations in counts/minute for tritium after injection into the tube and abdomen. As you can see, the tritium appeared almost immediately in the serum, reached its peak in 30 minutes, and then continuously decreased. The reabsorption of the tube is very similar to that of the peritoneum. Hardly any tritium activity was found in the tube after 14 days.

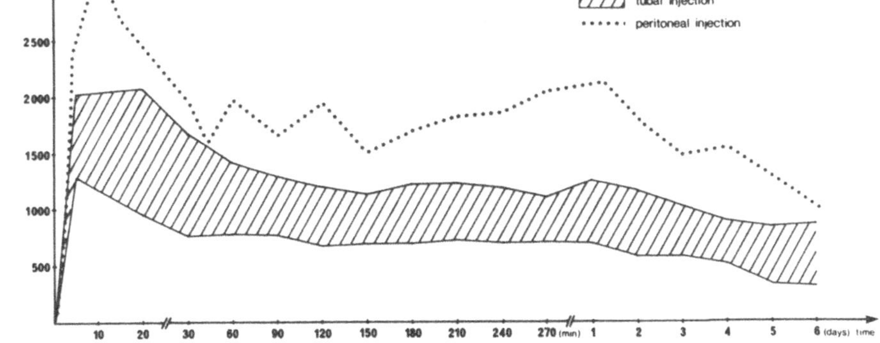

Figure 2 Serum tritium concentrations after injection into the hydrosalpinx and abdomen

hGH is reabsorbed by both the tube and the peritoneum more slowly and in smaller concentrations than was tritium. The maximum serum concentration was reached after 3 hours (Figure 3). The serum concentration started to decrease after 1 day. The residual activity for hGH was still very high at the end of the measurement period (3 days). The residual activity was about 20% (100 000 cpm).

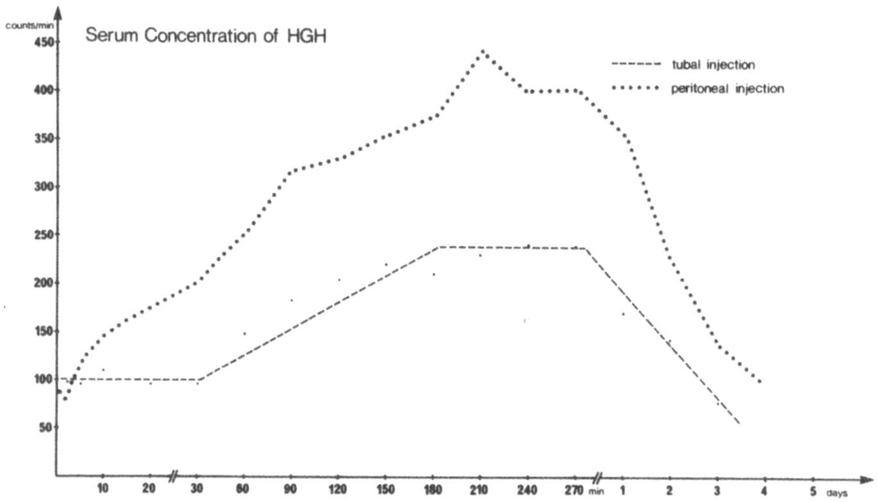

Figure 3 Serum [^{125}I]hGH concentrations after injection into the hydrosalpinx and abdomen

A similar pattern was found for albumin (Figure 4). A peak was finally reached 5–7 hours after a gradually increasing serum concentration. This concentration then decreased. The residual activity for radioactively labelled albumin in the tube was also still very high upon termination of the measurements.

Our findings can be summarized as follows:

(1) Water tritium was quickly reabsorbed out of the tube.
(2) The volume constancy of the hydrosalpinx can lead to a steady state due to the rapid exchange of H_2O.
(3) [^{125}I]albumin was reabsorbed slowly and in small concentrations out of the hydrosalpinx.
(4) [^{125}I]hGH was also reabsorbed in small concentrations (active transport?).

The reabsorption activity of the fallopian tube is comparatively similar to the peritoneum in the rabbit. We believe that the hydrosalpinx without an inflammatory reaction is no indication for surgical intervention.

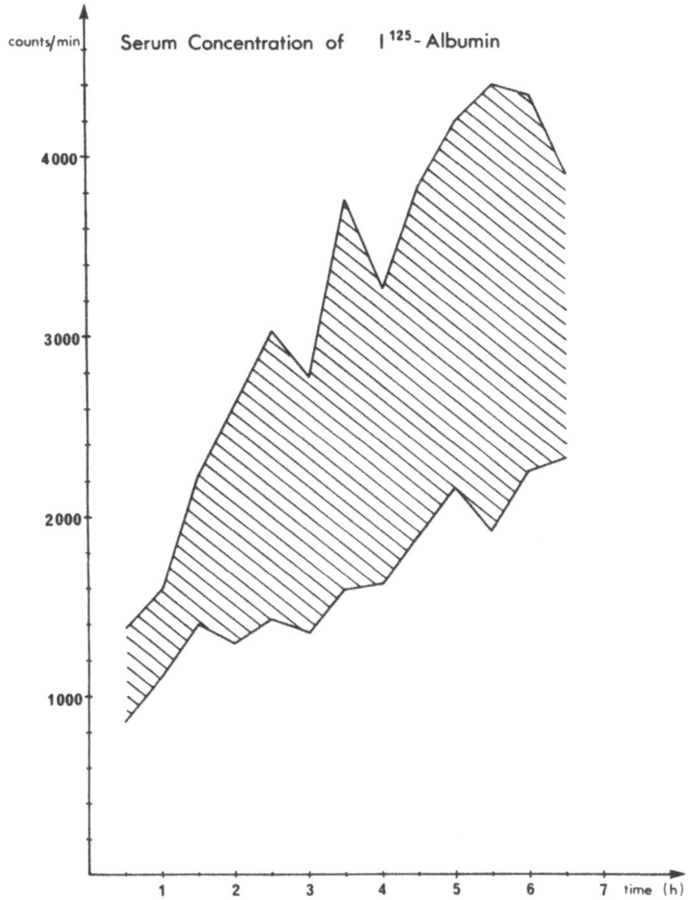

Figure 4 Serum [^{125}I]albumin concentrations after injection into the hydrosalpinx

Bibliography

1. Patek, E. and Nilsson, L. (1977). Hydrosalpinx simplex as seen by the scanning electron microscope. *Fertil. Steril.*, **28**, 962
2. Halbert, S. A. and Patton, D. L. (1981). Hydrosalpinx: Effect of oviductal dilatation on egg transport. *Fertil. Steril.*, **35**, 69
3. Vasquez, G., Oberti, C., Boeckx, W. and Winston, R. M. L. (1981). The evolution of experimentally, induced hydrosalpinges in rabbits. *Fertil. Steril.*, **35**, 342
4. Patton, D. L. and Halbert, S. A. (1981). Mechanically-induced hydrosalpinx: Long-term oviductal dilatation does not impair ciliary transport function. *Fertil. Steril.*, **36**, 808
5. Patton, D. L., Halbert, S. A. and San-Pin Wang, (1982). Experimental salpingitis in rabbits provoked by *Chlamydia trachomatis*. *Fertil. Steril.*, **37**, 691

Part I

Section 2
Microsurgical Techniques

3
Ultrastructural changes of the mucosa in rabbit fallopian tube after reanastomosis

S. NITSCHKE-DABELSTEIN, A. BÖGER, J. LÜTTGES and G. ZWIENS

Poly-Dioxanon (PDS, monofilament, Ethicon) and Polyglactin 910 (Vicryl, polyfilament absorbable suture, Ethicon) were used for reanastomosing rabbit fallopian tubes in order to investigate the tissue reaction to monofilament and polyfilament absorbable suture.

Eighteen female rabbits were laparotomized under general anaesthesia for unilateral reanastomosis after transsection of the tubal isthmus with microsurgical technique. Relaparotomy was performed either 6 weeks (10 animals) or 13–15 weeks (eight animals) later for dissection of the operated as well as the contralateral non-operated tubal isthmus. Comparative studies were done on tubes of non-operated animals.

The following ultrastructural changes of the mucosa could be outlined:

(1) Cytoplasmic blebs (Figure 1): segmentation from ciliated mucosa cells containing hyaloplasm, few ribosomes and fragments of microtubuli.
(2) Pathologically structured kinocilia presenting a disturbed arrangement of the microtubuli (Figure 1).
(3) Partial deciliation of the mucosal cells.
(4) Microglandular formations of various maturity.

Six weeks after reanastomosis mucosal folds of all fallopian tubes were covered by secretory and ciliated cells. Apical cell borders demonstrated sequestration of cytoplasmic blebs. Kinocilia were partly slender or distended and showed pathological internal structure. Long finger-like microvilli were dispersed in between. Suture fragments of both material were found in

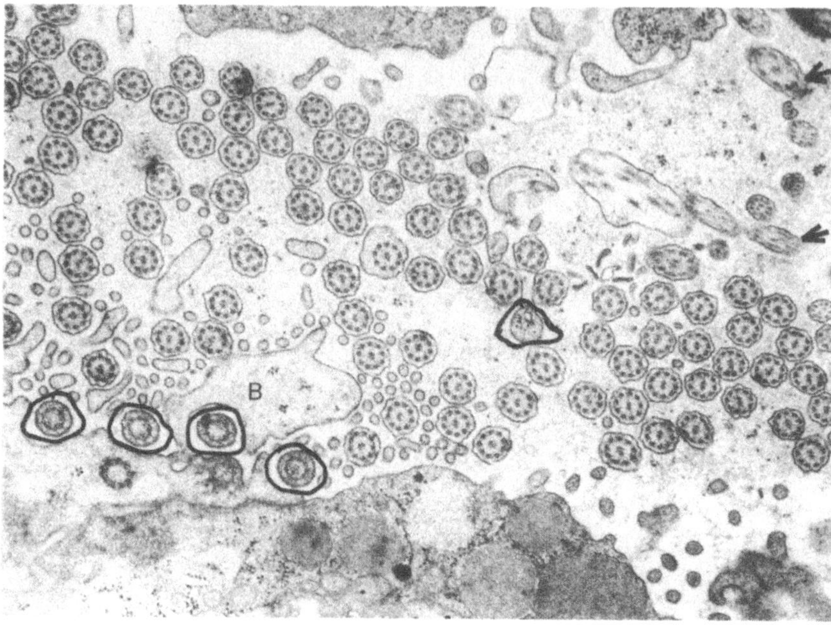

Figure 1 Transmission electronmicrograph of non-operated tube. B=Cytoplasmic blebs; ×16 100 pathologically structured kinocilia are encircled

Table 1 Ultrastructural changes of the rabbit tubal mucosa

Ultrastructural changes	*Reanastomosed tube*			*Contralateral non-operated tube*		
	PDS (*n*=5)	*Vicryl* (*n*=5)	*Total* (*n*=10)	*PDS* (*n*=5)	*Vicryl* (*n*=5)	*Total* (*n*=10)
			6 weeks after reanastomosis			
Cytoplasmic blebs	4	4	8	4	4	8
Pathologically structured kinocilia	2	1	3	2	0	2
Partial deciliation	3	2	5	2	0	2
			13–15 weeks after reanastomosis			
Cytoplasmic blebs	1	2	3	3	2	5
Pathologically structured kinocilia	1	0	1	1	0	1
Partial deciliation	1	0	1	3	2	5

macrophages. Significant differences depending on the kind of suture could not be evaluated.

13–15 weeks after reanastomosis similar ultrastructural changes were found. Above that at the basis of the mucosal folds narrow microglandular formations of various maturity appeared.

Contralateral non-operated tubal isthmi of both groups, 6 as well as 13–15 weeks after first laparotomy, demonstrated very similar lesions of the mucosal ultrastructure (Table 1). No such lesions were seen in fallopian tubes of the control group.

CONCLUSION

No significant differences in ultrastructural changes of the rabbit tubal mucosa after reanastomosis can be expected whether using monofilament or polyfilament absorbable suture. Changes of the mucosal ultrastructure after 6 as well as after 13–15 weeks demonstrated partial repair of the epithelium, best demonstrable in the ciliated cell. Similar lesions are described for the repaired hydrosalpinx by Petrucco and Tulsi[1].

Cytoplasmic blebs, as described, are observed in hypoxaemic and toxic damages of the liver, although not yet clearly interpreted in their function. Microglandulae might be a sign of an increased regeneration of the epithelium. A sympathetic-like lesion of the contralateral non-operated tube could be demonstrated.

The clinical relevance of this bilateral affection by unilateral operative procedure has to be further investigated.

Reference

1. Petrucco, O. M. and Tulti, R. S. (1981). Microsurgical reversal of the artificially induced hydrosalpinx in the rabbit-morphological studies. *N.Z.J. Obstet. Gynaecol.*, **21**, 159

4
Quantitative morphometrical and histopathological study in rabbit oviducts following microsurgical treatment

J. E. LÜTTGES, A. BÖGER, G. ZWIENS, U. PUDLO
and S. NITSCHKE-DABELSTEIN

Success of tubal reanastomosis in experimental studies has usually been confirmed by restoration of pathological lesions in the anastomosal site[1]. But little has been said about adjacent segments nor about alterations of the contralateral tube[2,3]. Therefore we decided to study animals with anastomosed and non-anastomosed contralateral oviducts in comparison with unoperated animals in order to examine whether alterations appear and whether they are effects of suture material and surgical procedure *per se*.

MATERIAL AND METHODS

In 21 rabbits weighing from 2000 to 2500 g isthmic reanastomosis was performed under microsurgical conditions with special avoidance of damage to blood vessels and peritoneum. A two-layer suture was placed excluding the mucosa. In 11 rabbits monofile Poly-p-dioxanon (PDS, Ethicon) was used and in a further 10 animals Vicryl (Ethicon) was used, both 8/0. At 6 weeks and 12 weeks respectively after operation the appropriate segments of 1.5 cm length were resected and immediately fixed in 4% formalin. The paraffin-embedded material was continuously cut into 5 μm sections and alternatively stained with haematoxylin-eosin and Elastica *v.* Gieson. For SEM, tissue was prepared according to the methods of Rosenbauer[4]. Morphometric investigations of 20 randomized sections of each tube were performed with Leitz A.S.M. and hook ocular, Leitz. SEM was done with a M7-SEM, ISI.

RESULTS

Six and 12 weeks postoperatively, only a slight inflammatory cellular infiltration was observed mainly in the subserous adipose tissue with an average of up to 11 lymphocytes and three macrophages in oviducts adjacent to the PDS anastomoses. Tissue adjacent to the Vicryl sutures showed a somewhat lower number with three lymphocytes and three macrophages at both time intervals. No inflammatory infiltration appeared on the contralateral oviducts nor in the controls.

Diameters of the muscularis on the anastomosed and on the non-anastomosed side revealed a significant difference from the non-laparatomized animals with values up to 220 μm compared with 127 μm of the control (Table 1). Thickening was mainly due to fibrosis documented by cell/stroma relation with an increase of stroma up to 20% in the anastomosed tube (Table 1). Even the contralateral oviduct showed a significant increase of fibrosis compared with controls. Neither suture material nor the time intervals influenced the degree of fibrosis.

At the bottom of the mucosal folds newly built, diffusely arranged microglands (Figure 1) appeared on the anastomosed and contralateral side (Table 2) with an increase especially in oviducts examined 12 weeks after operation.

By SEM, the oviduct epithelial layer was studied in another five operated animals, also in comparison with two controls.

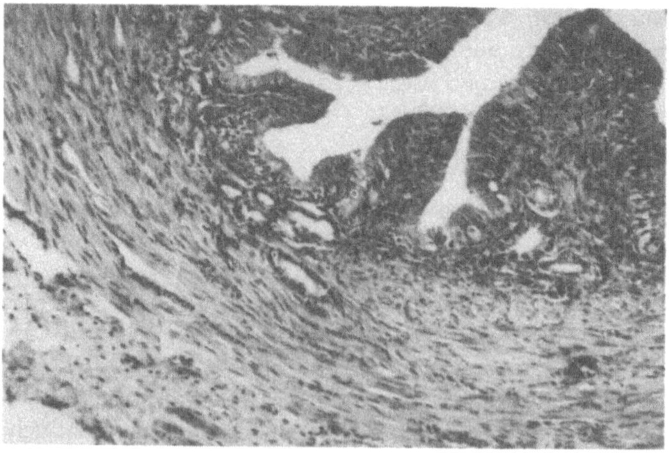

Figure 1 Microglands in the subepithelial stroma in a non-anastomosed oviduct, 12 weeks after operation. Haematoxylin and Eosin, ×16

Table 1 Diameter of the muscularis and cell-stroma relation as indicator of fibrosis

Group	*Diameter of muscularis* (μm) (mean ± sd)	*Significance of mean difference*	*Cell/stroma relation (% of cells)*	*Significance of mean difference*
Adjacent to PDS:				
Anastomosed ($n=4$) 6 weeks po	220 ± 38	NS to PDS	57	NS to Vicryl
Anastomosed ($n=4$) 12 weeks po	247 ± 39	nor to Vicryl	53	NS to Vicryl
Contralateral ($n=4$) 6 weeks po	185 ± 11	NS to anastomosed side	61	$p<0.05$ to anastomosed side
Contralateral ($n=4$) 12 weeks po	180 ± 9	NS to anastomosed side	61	$p<0.05$ to anastomosed side
Adjacent to Vicryl:				
Anastomosed ($n=4$) 6 weeks po	202 ± 26	NS to PDS nor to Vicryl	54	NS to PDS
Anastomosed (n=4) 12 weeks po	189 ± 16	NS to PDS nor to Vicryl	59	NS to PDS
Contralateral ($n=4$) 6 weeks po	184 ± 11	NS to anastomosed side	61	$p<0.05$ to anastomosed side
Contralateral ($n=4$) 12 weeks po	180 ± 9	NS to anastomosed side	61	$p<0.05$ to anastomosed side
Non-operated control ($n=6$)	127 ± 9	$p<0.01$ to non-anastomosed side $p<0.01$ to PDS $p<0.01$ to Vicryl	74	$p<0.01$ to non-anastomosed side $p<0.01$ to Vicryl $p<0.01$ to PDS

NS = Not significant; po = postoperatively.

Table 2 Microglands in subepithelial stroma: Average incidence, number and distribution

Group	*Cross-sections containing microglands (%)*	*No. (% of frequency)*		*Distribution (% of frequency)*	
		<5	*5–10*	*Diffuse*	*Local*
Adjacent to PDS:					
Anastomosed (n=4) 6 weeks po	32	52	38	18	32
Anastomosed (n=4) 12 weeks po	56	47	43	58	0
Contralateral (n=4) 6 weeks po	35	21	8	37	3
Contralateral (n=4) 12 weeks po	41	30	5	31	17
Adjacent to Vicryl:					
Anastomosed (n=4) 6 weeks po	31	52	41	37	23
Anastomosed (n=4) 12 weeks po	58	27	68	60	32
Contralateral (n=4) 6 weeks po	31	21	8	37	3
Contralateral (n=4) 12 weeks po	41	30	5	31	17
Non-operated control (n=6)	–	–	–	–	–

po = postoperatively.

The mucosa folds were regularly shaped on the anastomosed and contralateral side, and the relation of ciliated and secretory cells was normal. Single ciliated cells showed partial deciliation and shortening of ciliae (Figure 2).

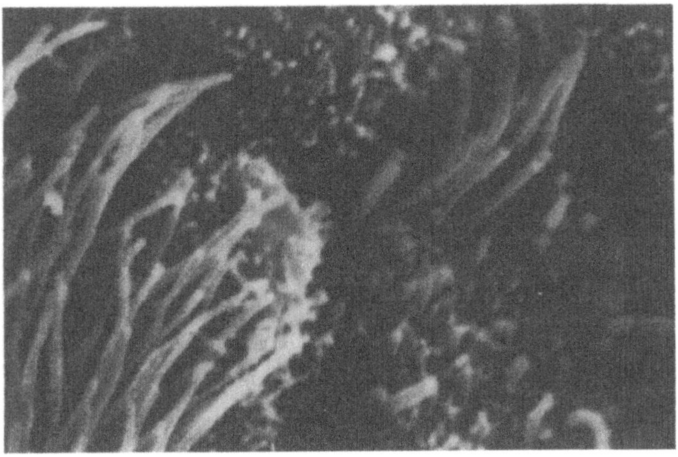

Figure 2 Partial deciliation and shortening of ciliae (at the right) in a non-anastomosed oviduct 6 weeks after operation. Scanning electron micrograph, ×10 000

Irregular vesicles demonstrating an increase of secretory activity appeared in ciliated and secretory cells.

DISCUSSION

Measurable pathological lesions in rabbit oviducts adjacent to an anastomose as well as on the contralateral side were found in contrast to results of Bernhardt-Huth[3]. The extent of these alterations, for example thickening of the muscularis, was nearly the same on both sides. There were no adhesions or damage of blood vessels that might explain these findings. Subepithelial microglands have never been reported before. They are not comparable with the pseudodiverticula[1,3,5] observed in the anastomosal site which are due to traumatically spread mucosa. Moreover, this aetiology would not explain the appearance of microglands on the contralateral side. Their increase after 12 weeks could be a sign of a chronic inflammatory reaction with epithelial hyper-regeneration. The importance of these glands remains to be investigated.

Although this was a small number of cases, it could be shown that any laparatomy causes remaining muscular fibrosis and epithelial lesions on the non-anastomosed oviduct which compare with alterations in tissue adjacent to the anastomoses.

References

1. Winston, R. L. M. (1975). Microsurgical reanastomosis of the rabbit oviduct and its functional and pathological sequelae. *Br. J. Obstet. Gynaecol.*, **82,** 513–22
2. Eddy, C. A., Flores, J. J., Archer, D. R. and Pauerstein, C. J. (1978). The role of cilia in fertility: An evaluation by selective microsurgical modification of the rabbit oviduct. *Am. J. Obstet. Gynecol.*, **132,** 814–20
3. Bernhardt-Huth, D., Frantzen, Ch. and Schlosser, H-W. (1981). Morphology of rabbit oviduct after microsurgical techniques for reanastomosis of the isthmus or ampulla. *Arch. Gynecol.*, **230,** 251
4. Rosenbauer, K. A. (1975). Die moderne Routine-präparation biologischer Objekte fur die Raster-elektronenmikroskopie. Paper presented at the *Technische Akademie Esslingen* 3–5 November
5. MacKay, E. V. and Khoo, S. K. (1972). Reactions in the rabbit fallopian tube after plastic reconstruction. II. Histopathology. *Fertil. Steril.*, **23,** 16

5
Reanastomosis of rabbit oviducts with monofilament and polyfilament absorbable sutures – a histological study

G. ZWIENS, A. BÖGER, J. LÜTTGES and S. NITSCHKE-DABELSTEIN

INTRODUCTION

In co-operation with the Department of Pathology of the University of Marburg we developed a useful animal model in order to test a new monofilament synthetic and resorbable suture made of polydioxanone. Its thickness is 8 × 0. We compared this suture with a polyfilament synthetic and resorbable suture made of polyglactin-910, which is known as Vicryl and is of the same thickness.

METHODS

After using halothane–nitrous-oxide gas as an anaesthetic a mid-line incision was made and 20 rabbit oviducts were reanastomosed in the isthmic region under microsurgical conditions. Table 1 shows the number of animals in the polyglactin and polydioxanone groups that were operated on and examined afterwards as well as the period after which the oviducts were removed.

We removed the oviducts of six animals belonging to the first group and eight animals belonging to the second one after 6–8 weeks whereas the oviducts of three animals of the first group and three animals belonging to the second group were removed after 12 weeks.

The anastomoses of 14 oviducts were examined by means of a light and transmission electron microscope whereas six oviducts were examined by means of a scanning electron microscope. We made sure beforehand that each of the oviducts was patent.

RESULTS

The results of our experiments are shown in Table 1. Those tubes that had been reanastomosed by means of a suture made of polyglactin showed – in one case out of three and in three cases out of four – a broadening of the mucosa folds; the oviducts that had been reanastomosed by using a polydioxanone-suture always showed remarkably broad mucosa folds. Concerning the frequency of the hyperplasia of mucosal glands we obtained the following results: three oviducts belonging to the polyglactin group showed this phenomenon whereas only two of the oviducts that had been reanastomosed by means of a polydioxanone suture showed broad mucosa folds.

Table 1 Frequency of histological changes of the mucosa after anastomosis

Group of rabbits	*No. in group*	*Mucosal folds broadening*	*Hyperplasia of mucosal glands*	*Submucosal fibrosis*
Polyglactin (12 weeks)	3	X	XX	XX
Polydioxanone (12 weeks)	3	XXX	XX	XXX
Polyglactin (6–8 weeks)	4	XXX	X	XXX
Polydioxanone (12 weeks)	4	XXXX	-	XXXX

A submucosal fibrosis was found with nearly all the examined oviducts.

Table 2 shows that, without exception, the oviducts developed fibrosis of the adventitia. Concerning the frequency of subserous muscle-bulging our results were quite different: only those oviducts that had been reanastomosed by using a polydioxanone suture showed subserous muscle bulging. To our surprise, we found a tissue reaction in some of the contralateral non-operated oviducts showing new formations of smooth muscle cells as previously described in the literature for the operated oviducts. Because of the rare occurrence of this phenomenon it has not been mentioned in the table.

Both after 6–8 and after 12 weeks remains of the suture that had been used were found in most of the oviducts within the cells. A macrophage is shown in Figure 1. It shows clearly that after 6 or 8 weeks the suture used in the operation can be found only within the cells. There are the remains of a polydioxanone suture in a 4000-fold magnification recognizable by its dark colour.

Table 2 Frequency of histological changes of the tubal wall after anastomosis

Group of rabbits	*No. in group*	*Subserous fibrosis*	*Subserous muscle-bulging*	*Suture remains*
Polyglactin (12 weeks)	3	XXX	X	XXX
Polydioxanone (12 weeks)	3	XXX	XX	XXX
Polyglactin (6–8 weeks)	4	XXXX	X	XX
Polydioxanone (6–8 weeks)	4	XXXX	XXXX	XXXX

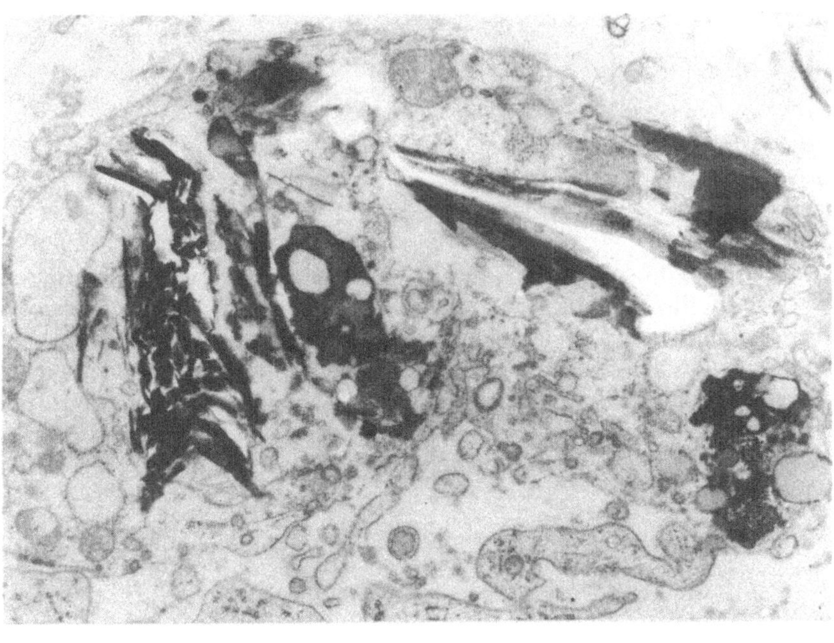

Figure 1 A macrophage with polydioxanone suture in it, ×4000

The ruptures of the sutures are the result of fixation. The mature collagen that has been developed by the fibroblast is shown in Figure 2. It indicates that the restoration of the tissue can be regarded as almost completed after 6 or 8 weeks. The picture was taken after reanastomosing a tube with a polydioxanone-suture by using an electron microscope. It shows the tube in a 5000-fold magnification. The fibres have all got the same thickness and are situated close to the cut fibroblasts.

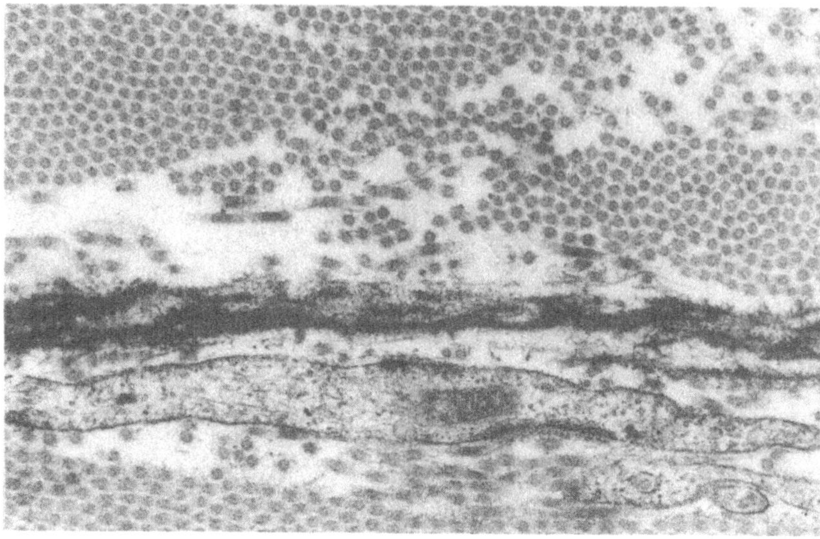

Figure 2 Mature collagen developed by a fibroblast. ×5000

DISCUSSION

It is interesting to compare the results we have obtained with those that are described in the literature concerning our subject. After reanastomosing several rabbit oviducts under microsurgical conditions we found a flat mucosa and thereby obtained the same results as have been worked out before on the basis of experiments by the team of Frantzen-Schlosser. Moreover, our slides showed newly developed smooth muscle cells near the serosa. Perhaps these newly developed muscle cells bring about a change in the motility of the tubal wall.

6
Conventional sutures *versus* fibrin glue in microsurgical anastomosis of reproductive tissue

D. SOJO, P. CUEVAS and J. CORTES

Microsurgery in gynaecology is a concept which represents much more than simple magnification. It requires an understanding of the oviduct physiology, very gentle tissue handling, scrupulous haemostasis, precise dissection, exact approximation of the tissue planes and the use of very fine suture materials. We have previously compared absorbable and non-absorbable microsutures in reproductive tissue and concluded that no significant functional differences were observed between oviduct reanastomosed with nylon and polyglactin suture[1].

On account of the success achieved by gluing nerve anastomoses[2] micro-vessels[3], vas deferens anastomoses[4] and rabbit fallopian tube[5] with a fibrinogen concentrate from human blood plasma, we wanted to introduce this technique in reproductive microsurgery.

We undertook the present study in order to examine the morphological characteristics of healing with and without the use of the fibrin glue. Animals were killed at various postoperative intervals after surgery. Histological reaction and adhesion formation were determined and compared.

MATERIALS AND METHODS

Twenty-eight female Wistar rats weighing between 200 and 250 g were used. The rats were anaesthetized with i.p. pentobarbital sodium. Under the operating microscope, the uterine horn was examined. After haemostasis of the uterine vessels, the horn was excised with microsurgical Vannas scissors. The two sutures were applied at 180 degrees (10.0 nylon monofilament with BV_2 needle, Ethicon), at the meso- and at the antimesenterical end. The same technique was employed in the left horn which served as a control. On the right one, the operation concluded with glue application. The abdominal wall was closed in two layers. As gluing material we used a fibrinogen concentrate produced from human blood plasma stabilized by the action of factor XIII; such a reaction was induced by addition of a thrombin solution (Tissucol, Immuno).

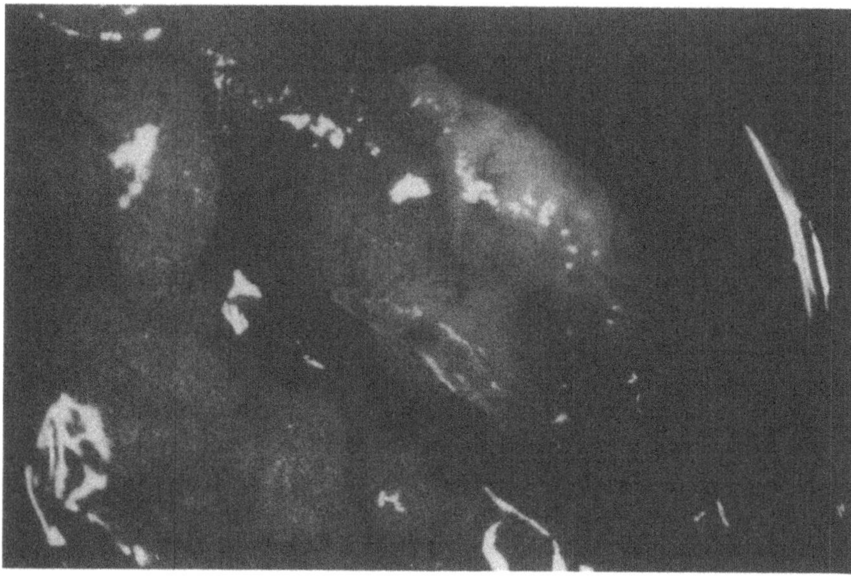

Figure 1 Glued end-to-end uterine horn anastomosis with two approximation sutures

At different postoperative times (24 h, 48 h and 8, 30, 60, 90 and 100 days), the animals were reoperated, adhesions were evaluated with the aid of the operating microscope according to Winston parameters and both horns were removed for histological study. The horn was excised above and below the anastomosis and fixed for electron microscopy by immersion in a mixture of glutaraldehyde and paraformaldehyde. Sections (1 μm thick) were cut with a glass knife and stained with toluidine blue for light microscopy. Half of each piece were prepared for SEM. All specimens were dehydrated in graded ethanols followed by acetone. They were dried from liquid CO_2 by the critical point method. Dried preparations were coated with gold and examined in a JEOL JSM 35C scanning electron microscope.

RESULTS

The results (Table 1) show that adhesions were almost always present to some degree in both horns.

Table 1 Adhesion formation in rat uterine horns

Group	*Approximation* (n=28)	*Approximation+fibrin glue* (n=28)
No microscopic adhesions	2	2
Mild (microscopic adhesions only)	10	11
Moderate adhesions (macroscopic horn)	14	13
Severe (horn and adjacent structures)	2	2

We did not find significant differences in adhesion formation between the approximated horns and the glued hornes. The majority of the animals showed abnormal mucosal fold pattern at the anastomotic site in both uterine horns. The lumina were slightly constricted in both uterine horns.

After application of the fibrin glue, the tissue reaction was moderate. A mild borderline infiltration of lymphocytes and polymorphonuclear leukocytes was observed at the fibrin cuff at 8 and 30 days.

Fibrin glue had been identified until 60 days after surgery, causing little connective tissue formation. Muscle continuity appeared relatively normal from 30 days onward, with minimal fibrous tissue replacement.

References

1. Sojo, D.J., Diaz Pardo, J. and Nistal, M. (1983). Histology and fertility after microsurgical anastomosis of the rabbit fallopian tube with nylon and polyglactin sutures. *Fertil. Steril.*, **39,** 707
2. Matras, H., Braun, F., Lassmann, H., Ammerer, H.P. and Mamoli, B. (1973). Plasma clot welding of nerves (experimental report). *J. Maxilo. Fac. Surg.*, **I,** 236
3. Kletter, G., Matras, H., Chiari, H., Dinges, N. and Witzmann, A. (1977). Comparative evaluation of conventionally sutured and clot-sutured microsurgical anastomosis. In Schmiedek, P. (ed.) *Microsurgery for Stroke.* pp. 149–53. (New York: Springer-Verlag)
4. Bach, D., Diestelmarer, W. and Weissbach, L. (1980). Animal experiments on reanastomosis of the vas deferens using fibrin glue. *Urol. Res.*, **8,** 29
5. Scheidel, P.H., Wallwiener, D.K., Weidemann, R.A. and Hepp, H.L., (1982). Experimental anastomosis of the rabbit fallopian tube using fibrin glue. *Fertil. Steril.*, **38,** 471

7
The tissue reaction to different kinds of suture material in the uterus and the oviduct of the rabbit

P. J. DÖRR, A. G. J. M. HANSELAAR, C. J. HERMAN, M. BOER-MEISEL and H. M. VEMER

INTRODUCTION

The tissue reaction of absorbable and non-absorbable suture material in the wall of the uterine horns and oviducts of the rabbit was studied.

The question was whether it is preferable to use non-absorbable suture material instead of hydrolytic absorbable suture material in gynaecological microsurgery.

Until now non-absorbable suture material has generally been used in gynaecological microsurgery, because it is supposed that the tissue reaction is less using non-absorbable suture material than when absorbable suture material is used, as with the absorption the tissue reaction would increase[1]. However, a literature study shows that the tissue reactions using hydrolytic absorbable and non-absorbable suture material are equal. The tissue reaction of hydrolytic absorbable suture material disappears with absorption while the tissue reaction of non-absorbable suture material persists[2-4].

MATERIALS AND METHODS

Six New Zealand White rabbits were used for the study. The suture materials were polyamide (Ethilon) and polypropylene (Prolene), both non-absorbable, and polyglactin 910 (Vicryl), hydrolytic absorbable, all 10×0 monofilament. Sutures were applied with an atraumatic BV-6 needle.

Under general anaesthesia a laparotomy by midline incision was performed. The suture material was placed in the wall of both uterine horns and in the wall of both oviducts with due regard to microsurgical principles: gentle tissue handling, irrigation of the operative field and use of a Zeiss OPMI-6 operating microscope. In one uterine horn the sutures were placed in a transverse, in the other in a longitudinal direction with the same procedure in both oviducts. The sutures were knotted three times in the usual way and the first knot was loosely tightened to prevent traction of the tissues. After 1, 3 and 8 weeks the uterine horns and the oviducts were removed, fixed in formaline 4% and examined histologically.

It was determined whether the suture material was macroscopically visible. Around every stitch as much tissue as possible was gathered, cut perpendicular to the stitch direction and separately embedded. Slides were made for histological evaluation, using haematoxylin and eosin stain.

Microscopically the solubility of the suture material and the kind and grade of the tissue reaction were examined. The kind of tissue reaction was classified as acute (presence of granulocytes), chronic (presence of lymphocytes, plasma cells, macrophages and giant cells) or late (increase in vessels and fibroblastic reaction). The grade of the tissue reaction was classified as absent, little, or strong.

RESULTS

Macroscopically polyglactin was not visible after 3 weeks. Microscopically the tissue reaction in all slides studied was chronic, with the presence of lymphocytes, plasma cells, macrophages and giant cells. The grade of the tissue reaction was generally little. There were no differences in tissue reaction in the three suture materials, in the uterus and oviduct, both in the transversely or longitudinally placed suture materials, after 1, 3 and 8 weeks. Microscopically polyglactin fragmented after 3 weeks without an increase in the tissue reaction.

DISCUSSION

Riddick *et al.*[5] compared polyglactic acid (Vicryl) and polyglycolic acid (Dexon), both hydrolytic absorbable suture materials, in rat uterine and abdominal wall tissues for inflammatory response. They found that the tissue reaction was significantly less in response to polyglactic acid (Vicryl) in both uterus and skin as compared with the response to polyglycolic acid (Dexon).

Dahlke *et al.*[3] compared polyamide (Ethilon) and polyglactin 910 (Vicryl), both monofilament 10×0, in vessel anastomoses in the rat and showed that polyglactin is absorbed after 8 weeks and that the tissue reaction disappeared after 10 weeks, while the tissue reaction after anastomoses using Ethilon persisted.

Ippisch *et al.*[4], using the same suture materials in vessel and nerve anastomoses in the rat, found that the tissue reaction after anastomoses with polyglactin disappeared after 10–12 weeks.

Our results are in accordance with the literature. There were no differences in tissue reaction in the three suture materials studied. After fragmentation of polyglactin there was no increase in tissue reaction. It is to be expected that with the absorption of polyglactin the tissue reaction will disappear.

Our study shows that hydrolytic absorbable suture material can be used in gynaecological microsurgery.

Acknowledgements

The suture materials were kindly provided by Ethicon, Hamburg, West Germany.

References

1. Winston, R. M. L. (1980). Microsurgery of the fallopian tube: From fantasy to reality. *Fertil. Steril.*, **34**, 521
2. Blomstedt, B. (1977). Experiences with polyglactin 910 (Vicryl) in general surgery. *Acta Chir. Scand.*, **143**, 259
3. Dahlke, H., Dociv, N. and Thurau, K. (1979). Synthetisches resorbierbares und synthetisches nicht resorbierbares Nahtmaterial in der mikrovaskulären Chirurgie. *Handchirurgie*, **11**, 3
4. Ippisch, A., Wriedt-Lübbe, I., Duspiva, W. and Blümel, G. (1980). Mikrochirurgische Nerven- und Gefässnähte mit resorbierbarem Nahtmaterial. *Z. Plastische Chir.*, **4**, 2
5. Riddick, J. H., De Crazia, C. T. and Maenza, R. M. (1977). Comparison of polyglactic and polyglycolic acid sutures in reproductive tissue. *Fertil. Steril.*, **28**, 1220

8
Prevention of adhesions and restoring patency during oviduct anastomosis in rabbits: microscope *versus* loupes

H. M. VEMER, W. BOECKX and I. A. BROSENS

INTRODUCTION

Prevention of adhesions is a major challenge in tubal surgery. Fibrinous material, deposited on the peritoneal surface, may either be reabsorbed completely or turn into fibrous adhesions by the ingrowth of capillaries and fibroblasts. The crucial question is what determines the fate of the fibrinous material. Although many regimens were tried to prevent adhesion formation, gentle tissue handling still appears to be the most rational approach to avoid ischaemia of the peritoneal surface.

Khoo and Mackay[1] reported that 53% of their rabbits had patent oviducts after macrosurgical anastomosis. Paterson and Wood reported more than 90% patent oviducts in rabbits after microsurgical anastomosis[2]. However, Hedon *et al.*[3] reached almost the same results using a loupe.

In this study we investigated the effect of the use of a microscope or the use of loupes by studying the adhesion formation and the patency rates after oviduct anastomosis in rabbits.

MATERIALS AND METHODS

Sixteen female, adult, non-pregnant New Zealand White rabbits were used.

After laparotomy by midline incision, under general anaesthesia, the right oviduct was cut with scissors. After scrupulous haemostasis with bipolar coagulation, anastomosis was performed using Keeler loupes (×4 magnification and focal distance 28 cm). Anastomosis was made in two layers: muscularis to muscularis and serosa to serosa, trying to avoid the mucosa. During the same anaesthesia, the left oviduct was also cut with scissors. After scrupulous bipolar haemostasis a two-layer anastomosis was made, this time using a Zeiss OPMI-6 operating microscope at magnification 2.4×–16×. In half the animals the microscope was used first, and in half the loupes.

All operations were performed by the first author using microsurgical techniques and 10/0 nylon. 15 ml sodium chloride 0.9% was instilled intraperitoneally before closing the abdomen. 2 weeks later, a second laparotomy was performed to check the anastomoses by injecting methylene blue into the uterus. The adhesions were then classified according to Winston[4]:

(1) Absent (no microscopic adhesions).
(2) Mild (microscopic adhesions only).
(3) Moderate (macroscopic adhesions, oviduct only).
(4) Severe (oviduct and adjacent structures).

Statistical analysis was performed with a χ^2 test.

RESULTS

The degree of adhesion formation after anastomosis with the aid of a loupe or with the aid of an operating microscope is shown in Table 1. The difference between the degree of adhesion formation in the two groups was statistically significant ($p < 0.05$).

Table 1 Adhesion formation after oviduct anastomosis under a loupe and under an operating microscope

Adhesions	*Loupe*	*Microscope*
None	6	11
Mild	4	4
Moderate	5	1
Severe	1	0

Table 2 Oviduct patency after oviduct anastomosis under a loupe or under an operating microscope

Oviduct	*Loupe*	*Microscope*
Patent	10	16
Non-patent	6	0

The patency rates after anastomosis are shown in Table 2. This difference was also statistically significant ($p < 0.01$).

DISCUSSION

Adhesion prevention is still a major goal in fertility surgery. Rough handling of the tissues, resulting in ischaemic or necrotic tissue, is probably responsible for a great deal of adhesion formation. Our data indicate that adequate magnification can prevent tissue damage and thus lead to adhesion prevention.

Furthermore, we showed that adequate magnification with an operating microscope is necessary to distinguish serosa, muscularis and mucosa in order to obtain patency after oviduct anastomosis.

Our data support the view that microsurgery still forms the best way to perform tubal surgery[5].

References

1. Khoo, S.K. and Mackay, E.V. (1972). Reactions in rabbit fallopian tube after plastic reconstruction. *Fertil. Steril.*, **23**, 201
2. Paterson, P. and Wood, C. (1974). The use of microsurgery in the reanastomosis of the rabbit fallopian tube. *Fertil. Steril.*, **25**, 757
3. Hedon, B., Wineman, M. and Winston, R.M.L. (1980). Loupes or microscope for tubal anastomosis? *Fertil, Steril.*, **34**, 264
4. Winston, R.M.L. (1975). Microsurgical reanastomosis of the rabbit oviduct and its functional and pathological sequelae. *Br. J. Obstet. Gynaecol.*, **82**, 513
5. Vemer, H.M., Boeckx, W. and Brosens, I. (1982). The use of dextrans for the prevention of postoperative peritubal adhesions in rabbits. *Br. J. Obstet. Gynaecol.*, **89**, 473

9
Inhibition of peritoneal adhesion formation by colchicine

M. GRANAT, I. TUR-KASPA, E. ZYLBER-KATZ
and J. G. SCHENKER

INTRODUCTION

Despite a substantial amount of research, there is no mode of therapy that satisfactorily prevents the formation of postoperative peritoneal adhesions. Therefore, the search for a reliable prophylactic agent continues. Colchicine, a microtubular-disruptive drug, may be beneficial owing to its inhibitory effects on processes in the pathogenesis of peritoneal adhesions, such as: (1) inhibition of histamine secretion from mast cells[1], (2) an antimititic effect[2] and (3) inhibition of synthesis and secretion of collagen from fibroblasts[3-5]. Much experience has been gained from the safe, long-term use of colchicine in familial mediterranean fever (FMF)[6]. This study has been carried out in an attempt to verify our previous encouraging results indicating the decrease in adhesion formation after colchicine administration[7].

MATERIALS AND METHODS

Induction of adhesions

Seventy-two white female Sabra rats weighing 180–200 g were anaesthetized with ether and their skin was shaved and cleansed. A 4 cm lower midline incision was made in the abdominal wall. A method of multiple trauma was used to induce adhesions, in which the extent of trauma made as uniform as possible:

(1) The dorsal surfaces of the uterine horns were abraded with a scalpel blade until macroscopic bleeding ensued.
(2) The caecum was delivered from the wound, and its surface rubbed briskly with a sterile gauze until petechial haemorrhages appeared.
(3) The ileum, 10 cm from the ileocaecal junction, was abraded with a scalpel at three 1 cm segments, separated by intervals of 1 cm. No antibiotics were administered. The abdominal incision was closed in two layers with 3–0 catgut sutures.

Drug administration

After operation the rats were randomly divided into three groups, each comprising 24 animals and assigned as (1) colchicine, (2) dexamethasone and (3) control groups. Rats in the colchicine group received 14 daily intramuscular injections of 50 μg colchicine, dissolved in 0.5 ml sterile water. Rats of the dexamethasone group received intramuscular injections of 0.1 mg dexamethasone, in 0.5 ml normal saline, four times daily, to a total of nine doses. Rats of the control group were injected with 0.5 ml normal saline once a day for 14 days.

Evaluation of adhesions

4 weeks after laparotomy all the rats were killed, their abdominal cavities were exposed and the number and degree of adhesions recorded. To avoid bias, the animals were coded and examined without knowledge of whether they were from a study or control group. In addition to the number of adhesions, a grading scale of 0–4 was applied to record their severity based on quality and distribution:

Grade 0 - no adhesions.
Grade 1 - thin, filamentous, easily separated adhesions.
Grade 2 - thick adhesions in a limited area.
Grade 3 - widespread, thick adhesions.
Grade 4 - grade 3 plus adherence of visceral organs.

The average double-product of the number of adhesions multiplied by their grading was used as an estimate of the severity of adhesions.

Mann–Whitney U tests and χ^2 tests were used for statistical analysis.

RESULTS

The dosage of colchicine was chosen after a pilot study where plasma colchicine concentration was measured in four groups of rats 2 hours after intramuscular injection of different doses of colchicine. A linear correlation was found between the dose and plasma level. A daily dose of 50 μg rendered plasma levels in the range of that observed in FMF patients under continuous colchicine treatment (2–16 $ng\,ml^{-1}$)[8]. The dosage of dexamethasone was equivalent, on a weight-to-weight basis, to that given to women following pelvic surgery[9].

Since a very mild degree of adhesion-formation is usually insignificant with regard to fertility, we have chosen the criteria of at least two grade 3 adhesions in a rat as an indicator of marked adhesion formation. This occurred in only 18.2% of the colchicine group, as compared with 40.9% of the control group ($p < 0.02$). When the criterion of severity of adhesions was changed to at least three grade 3 adhesions, the difference between these groups became even more significant (9.1% *vs.* 59%; $p < 0.001$). The difference between the dexamethasone and control groups was not significant applying both criteria.

DISCUSSION

Peritoneal adhesions are the consequence of an inflammatory reaction and a healing process following damage to the peritoneum, such as trauma during surgery[10]. Histamine secretion from mast cells, fibroblast proliferation and secretion of collagen are involved in their pathogenesis[11,12]. Hence colchicine has been investigated as a potential anti-adhesion-formation agent, owing to its antihistamine[1] and antimitotic effects[2] as well as to its inhibitory effect on collagen synthesis and secretion[3–5]. Colchicine administered intramuscularly to rats in a dose that rendered plasma levels in a range similar to that observed in FMF patients under long-term therapy has been shown in this study to reduce significantly the severity of adhesion formation compared with that found in dexamethasone-treated and untreated groups of rats. Individual variations observed within each group could originate in part from the unavoidable subjective evaluation of the severity of adhesions after treatment. They may also be analogous to the differences, hitherto unpredictable, of healing patterns of the peritoneum following surgical trauma among human subjects.

Similar results were previously obtained following intraperitoneal administration of suprapharmacological doses of colchicine (0.4 $mg\,kg^{-1}$) in rats for 3 weeks, with no detectable untoward effects[7]. Side-effects of colchicine rarely occur and are mild and tolerable[6], provided that over-dosage is avoided. We are currently investigating the value of this convenient and relatively safe therapy in primates as a potential substitute for the commonly used dexamethasone.

References

1. Lagunoff, D. and Chi, E. Y. (1976). Effect of colchicine on rat mast cell. *J. Cell Biol.*, **71**, 182
2. Brues, A. M. and Cohen, A. (1936). Effects of colchicine and related substances to cell division. *Biochem. J.*, **30**, 1363
3. Diagelmann, R. F. and Peterkofsky, B. (1972). Inhibition of collagen secretion from bone and cultured fibroblasts by microtubular disruptive drugs. *Proc. Natl. Acad. Sci. USA*, **69**, 892
4. Erlich, H. P., Ross, R. and Bornstein, P. (1974). Effects of antimicrotubular agents on the secretion of collagen: a biochemical and morphological study. *J. Cell. Biol.*, **62**, 390
6. Levy, M. and Eliakim, M. (1977). Long-term colchicine prophylaxis in familial mediterranean fever. *Br. Med. J.*, **ii**, 808
7. Shapiro, I., Granat, M. and Sharf, M. (1982). The effect of intraperitoneal colchicine on formation of peritoneal adhesions in the rat. *Arch. Gynecol.*, **231**, 227
8. Zylber-Katz, E., Ehrenfeld, M., Levy, M. and Eliakim, M. (1982). Plasma colchicine concentration in patients with recurrent polyserositis (familial mediterranean fever) on long-term prophylaxis. *Arthr. Rheum.*, **25**, 227
9. Granat, M., Schenker, J. G., Mor-Yosef, S., Rosenkovitch, E., Cano Castellanos, R. and Galili, U. (1983). Effects of dexamethasone on proliferation of autologous fibroblasts and on the immune-profile in women undergoing pelvic surgery for infertility. *Fertil. Steril.*, **39**, 180
10. Pfeffer, W. H. (1980). Adjuvants in tubal surgery. *Fertil. Steril.*, **33**, 245
11. Ellis, H. (1971). The cause and prevention of post-operative intraperitoneal adhesions. *Surg. Gynecol. Obstet.*, **133**, 497
12. Milligon, D. W. and Raftery, A. T. (1974). Observations on the pathogenesis of peritoneal adhesions: a light and electron microscopical study. *Br. J. Surg.*, **61**, 271

10
Prevention of re-formation of pelvic adhesions by 'barrier' methods

M. YEMINI, A. MESHORER, Z. KATZ, D. ROZENMAN
and M. LANCET

The postoperative formation or re-formation of pelvic adhesions still represents a major problem contributing to the relatively poor results obtained in infertility surgery. Chemical methods using heparin, trypsin, streptokinase and dextran have been employed in an attempt to diminish the occurrence of adhesions[1,2]. Several authors have used 'barrier' methods to cover the injured area, thereby preventing the formation of adhesions. Amnion, silicone and Surgicel have been used for this purpose, with varying results[3–5]. We report here on the effect of silicone sheeting and of Surgicel in preventing the re-formation of pelvic adhesions in rabbits.

MATERIALS AND METHODS

Animals and operative procedures

Twenty-five female rabbits (3–4 kg in weight) underwent laparotomy under general anaesthesia. The laparotomy was performed through a lower abdominal midline incision using a sterile technique. The uterine horns on each side were subjected to a standardized symmetrical injury by cautery. The injured area was 1 cm long, starting at the tubo-uterine junction and enveloping the uterine horns. No attempt at haemostasis was made. 10 days later the animals were re-operated and adhesions were scored and lysed. In ten animals (group A) the lesions on one side were covered with a silicone sheet

(Silastic, medical grade silicone elastomer, 1.8 mm (0.07 in) reinforced sheet (Dow Corning)), and in ten others (group B) they were covered with Surgicel (Surgicel, sterilized oxidized cellulose (B.P. Ethicon)). The uterine horn side on which lesions were to be covered was chosen randomly by an investigator who was not involved in the study. The segments of silicone and of Surgicel were 2×3 cm in size and were placed over the injured areas with interrupted 5–0 Prolene sutures. The contralateral uterine horn in each animal served as an internal control group. Five animals (group C) in whom no barrier was used served as an external control group. During a third operation 10 days later the silicone segments in group A animals were removed.

The rabbits were killed and examined for pelvic adhesions 10 days after the third operation in group A and 10 days after the second operation in groups B and C.

The adhesions were scored according to the following classification (modified from that of Knightly *et al.*[6]):

Grade 0 – Absence of adhesions.
Grade 1 – A single filmy, easily separated adhesion.
Grade 2 – Extensive, filmy adhesions.
Grade 3 – A single dense adhesion requiring sharp dissection.
Grade 4 – More than one dense adhesion.

During the last operation on each rabbit, tissue from the traumatized area of both uterine horns was removed for histological examination.

Statistics – The data were analysed by the Mann–Whitney U test and by the Wilcoxon test.

RESULTS

One animal from group A and one from group B died under anaesthesia during the second operation and were excluded from the study. At the third operation the silicone segment was found to be covered on the surface facing the peritoneum with a delicate membrane tissue which was easily removed together with the silicone segment without dissection.

After the first operation, no significant differences in adhesions score were noted either between or within the groups (Table 1). In group A, on the side which was subsequently covered, the mean score was 2.9±0.8, and on the contralateral side the mean was 2.8±0.8. In group B the mean scores were 2.4±1.0 and 2.3±0.5 respectively, and the mean score for group C was 2.4±1.0. Furthermore no significant differences in re-formation of adhesions were noted between group C (mean 2.5±1.0) and the internal control sides of group A (mean 2.5±1.3) or of group B (mean 2.5±1.13); these results, moreover, were not significantly different from the mean adhesion scores following the first operation in all groups.

Table 1 Mean (±SE) adhesions score

		Adhesions score following diathermy		*Adhesions score following lysis*	
Group	*No. of animals*	*Treated side*	*Internal control*	*Treated side*	*Internal control*
A	9	2.9±0.8*	2.8±0.8	1.4±1.5*†	2.5±1.3
B	9	2.4±1.0	2.3±0.5	3.8±0.4†‡¶	2.5±1.1¶
C	5	2.4±1.0		2.5±1.0†	

Difference between means significant: *$p<0.006$; † $p<0.02$; ‡ $p<0.009$; ¶ $p<0.01$.

In group A on the treated side, adhesion re-formation was reduced (mean 1.4±1.5). The degree of reduction was highly significant in comparison with that on the same side following the first operation ($p<0.006$) and with the re-formation of adhesions in the external control ($p<0.02$), but only of borderline significance in comparison with the re-formation of adhesions in the internal control ($p<0.07$). In group B, on the other hand, the degree of re-formation of adhesions on the treated side was significantly increased (mean 3.8±0.4) in comparison with that after the first operation ($p<0.009$), and with those of the internal ($p<0.01$) and the external controls ($p<0.02$).

Histological examination of the membrane covering the silicone segment revealed a thin sheet of fibrin with few fibroblasts and early capillary proliferation. Microscopic examination of the treated uterine horns in group A carried out during the final operation revealed only a few inflammatory cells and almost complete healing of the injured area.

In group B, microscopically small residua of Surgicel were found at postmortem. They were surrounded by fibroblast and inflammatory cells in a typical foreign body reaction.

DISCUSSION

The results of our study indicate that Surgicel is ineffective in preventing the re-formation of adhesions, and may even promote their formation. Silicone, on the other hand, has been found to be uniquely inert when implanted in the abdominal cavity[7]. This was confirmed by our histological examination of the injured area in group A. Others have suggested that silicone, when used as a synthetic barrier, acts as foreign body[5]; however, the silk sutures used by these authors may have promoted adhesion formation, since silk is known to cause tissue reaction. Cook *et al.*[8] reported a significant reduction in adhesion formation when silicone film was used.

Our results suggest that silicone sheeting is an effective barrier method for preventing the re-formation of pelvic adhesions. Although the reduction in adhesion formation was only of borderline significance when compared with that of the internal control, it was highly significant when compared with that of the external control or with initial adhesion formation on the same side. These findings, together with the lack of significant differences in the degrees of adhesion formation and re-formation either between or within the external and internal controls, support the conclusion that silicone is an effective barrier and can be used in preventing the re-formation of adhesions. Further research is necessary in order to determine the exact time at which the silicone should be removed from the pelvis, as well as its effectiveness when used in conjunction with other materials such as dextran.

References

1. Stangel, C.J. and Gomel, V. (1980). Postoperative adhesions: Etiology, prevention and therapy. *Clin. Obstet. Gynecol.*, **23**, 1213
2. Seitz, H.M., Schenker, J.G., Epstein, S. and Garcia, C.R. (1973). Postoperative intraperitoneal adhesions: A double-blind assessment of their prevention in the monkey. *Fertil. Steril.*, **24**, 935
3. Kubanyi, A. (1947). Prevention of peritoneal adhesions by transplantation of amnion. *Br. Med. J.*, **2**, 55
4. Larsson, B., Nisell, H. and Granberg, I. (1978). Surgicel - an absorbable hemostatic material in prevention of peritoneal adhesions in rats. *Acta Chir. Scand.*, **144**, 375
5. Soules, M.R., Dennis, L., Bosarge, A. and Moore, D.E. (1982). The prevention of postoperative pelvic adhesions: An animal study comparing barrier methods with dextran 70. *Am. J. Obstet. Gynecol.*, **143**, 829
6. Knightly, J.J., Agostino, D. and Clifton, E.E. (1962). The effect of fibrinolysin and heparin on the formation of peritoneal adhesions. *Surgery*, **52**, 250
7. Spiers, A.C. and Blocksma, R. (1963). New implantable silicon rubbers. *Plast. Reconstruct. Surg.*, **31**, 106
8. Cook, G.B. (1964). The silicone serosal interface. I. Abatement of talc adhesions in dogs. *Surgery*, 55, 268

Part II

Tubo-Uterine Infection

11
Scanning electron microscopic studies on the changes of the oviduct due to ageing, menstrual cycle, pregnancy and inflammation

T. HASHIMOTO, S. KAWAKAMI, M. MORISADA, T. FUJIWARA and R. IIZUKA

MATERIALS AND METHODS

Specimens used in this study were obtained from the ampulla of the oviducts of 54 human females during the following periods: fetal period, prepuberty, puberty, reproductive, menopausal and postmenopausal periods. The oviducts were excised and rapidly immersed in 2.5% glutaraldehyde solution for 1 h and phosphate buffer solution for 6 h and the tissues were postfixed in 1% OsO_4 solution for 1 h. After dehydration with graded concentrations of alcohol, they were placed in 100% amyl acetate and critical-point dried. They were mounted on the column and coating with carbon and gold, and examined by JSM 35 C electron microscope.

RESULTS

Fetal period – The presence of cilia was clearly recognized in the oviduct of the 20-week-old fetus (Figure 1).

Prepuberty – We could distinguish ciliated cells from secretory cells in the oviduct of the 11-month-old child. Developed cilia as well as developed microvilli were observed in the 10-year-old girl before menarche.

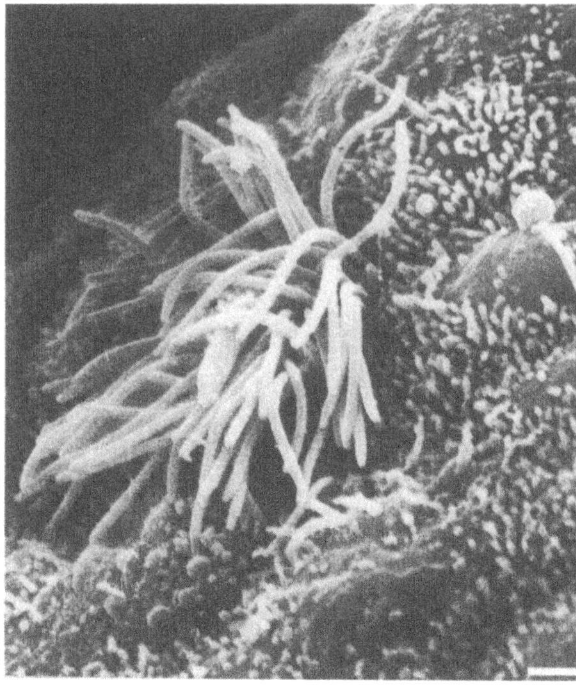

Figure 1 SEM of the oviduct of the 20-week-old fetus. ×12 000

Puberty – Ciliated cells with well-developed cilia and secretory cells with well-developed microvilli were found in the oviduct of the 14-year-old girl, 1 year after menarche.

Reproductive period – During menstruation and the follicular phase secretory cells appeared flat; contrastingly, during the ovulatory and luteal phases, they became swollen, which was suggestive of secretory activity. And the swelling of secretory cells and their secretory activity were observed in the pregnant cases. Ciliated cells, however, did not show remarkable changes (Figures 2 and 3).

Menopause and post-menopause – Secretory cells became flat and polygonal, also the contours of the cells became indistinctive, and no secretory activity was found. Cilia were well preserved in a 75-year-old woman (Figure 4).

In hydrosalpinx cases – Both secretory cells and ciliated cells were destroyed; in addition, desquamation of the epithelium was found.

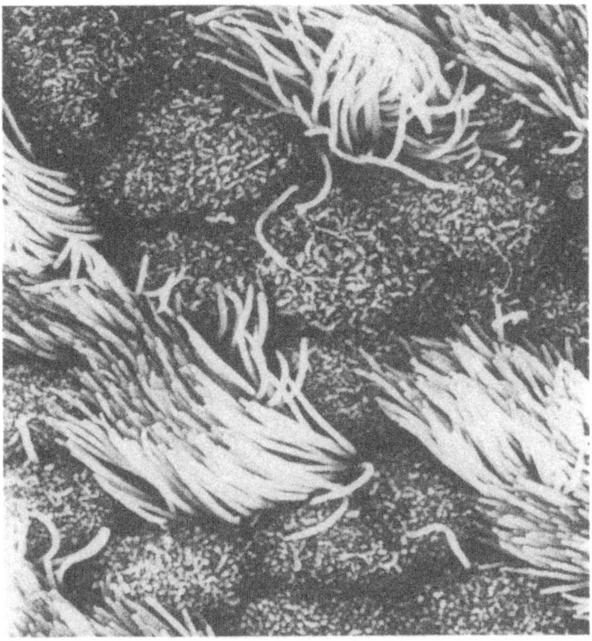

Figure 2 SEM of the oviduct during the follicular phase. ×6000

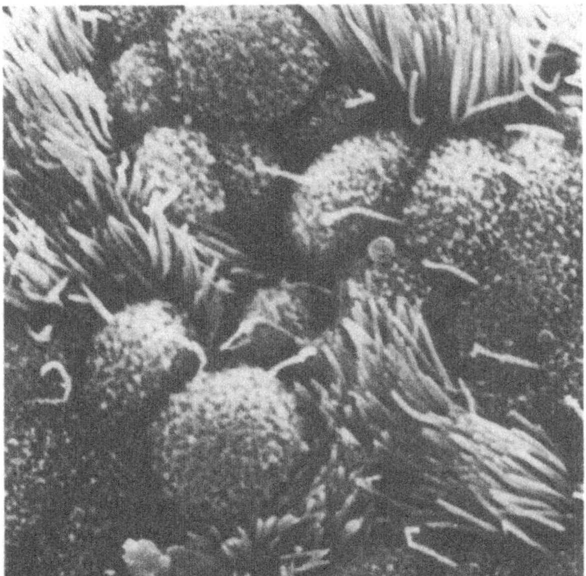

Figure 3 SEM of the oviduct during the luteal phase. ×6000

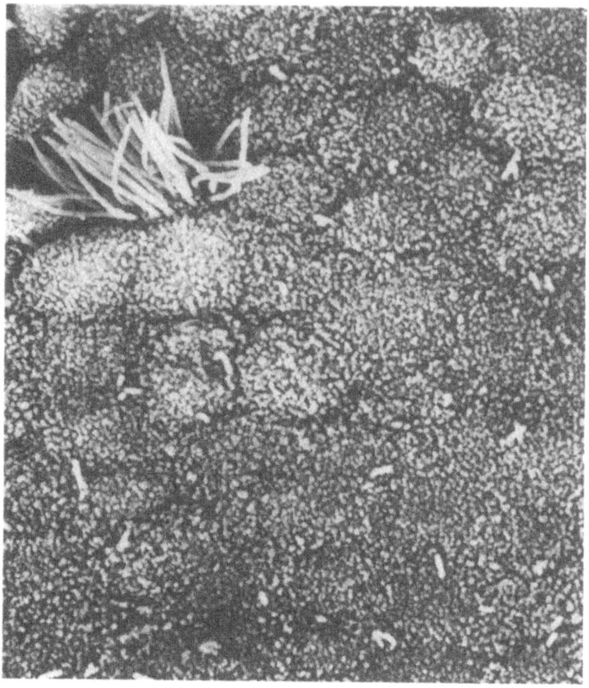

Figure 4 SEM of the oviduct of the 75-year-old woman. ×6000

DISCUSSION

As described above, the presence of cilia is recognized during the fetal period. Hashimoto *et al.*[1] and Patek *et al.*[2] examined the oviducts from fetuses at midgestation in TEM and in SEM. They have been able to identify both ciliated cells and non-ciliated cells. Komatsu and Fujita[3] have reported that the differentiation of the ciliated cells in the mouse oviduct began 5 days after birth, and features of ciliogenesis were found up to 5–10 days after birth. They suggested that the effect of ovarian hormones on ciliogenesis was not so important. In the reproductive period, ciliated cells show no particular changes. Komatsu and Fujita[3] observed that ciliated cells in the mouse oviduct undergo no cyclic changes even at reproductive age. In the post-menopausal period, secretory cells become flat and polygonal; also the contours of the cells become indistinctive, and no finding of secretory activity can be seen. On the other hand, even 30 years after menopause, cilia are well preserved and deciliation is not found. And cilia are destroyed in chronic inflammation such as hydrosalpinx cases, but the maintenance of cilia is not affected by ovarian hormones.

We agree with previous authors that ovarian hormones have an influence on the secretory cells in the ampulla of the human oviduct but ciliated cells are refractory to ovarian hormones in morphological changes.

References

1. Hashimoto, M. *et al.* (1962). Electron microscopic studies on the epithelial cells of the human fallopian tube, report I. *J. Jpn. Obstet. Gynecol. Soc.*, **9**, 202–9
2. Patek, E., Nilsson, E. and Johannisson, E. (1972). Scanning electron microscopic study of the human fallopian tube. Report II. Fetal life, reproductive life and postmenopause. *Fertil. Steril.*, **23**, 719–33
3. Komatsu, M. and Fujita, H. (1978). Electron-microscopic studies on the development and ageing of the oviduct epithelium of mice. *Anat. Embryol.*, **152**, 243–59

12
Chronic histological inflammation and *Chlamydia trachomatis* in women selected for tuboplasties

J. DE BRUX, J. HENRY-SUCHET, P. BUSSIERE, A. ARDOIN, F. CATALAN, D. SERFATY and V. LOFFREDO

Our previous work[1] has shown that *Chlamydia trachomatis* (CT), evidenced either by laparoscopic-positive cultures or by positive serodiagnosis, is significantly related to tubal factors of sterility, most of the women studied having no past history of salpingitis. In addition, our results showed that in such cases this infection can be found more frequently in women who had laparoscopic signs of chronic inflammation (that we called cases of 'viscous pelvis') than in women who presented no such signs.

The objective of this work is to carry out on a new series of women with tubal sterility a complete bacteriological, cytological and histological study. The investigation extends our previous findings concerning CT as a major agent of tubal sterility and correlates CT infection with a chronic evolutive inflammatory condition, assessed either macroscopically or by histological or cytological examinations.

MATERIALS AND METHODS

From October 1981 to December 1982, 74 women undergoing laparoscopy for sterility problems of obstructive origin (tubal stenosis or obstruction and/or periadnexal adhesions) had a complete bacteriological study of their lower genital tracts, their higher pelvic tracts (liquid from the Pouch of

Douglas or from hydrosalpinges, micro-biopsies of the fimbria and of adhesions) together with a cytological and histological study of the same samples. They also had a serological study for CT.

The techniques for samples and cultures for aeroanaerobics, CT and mycoplasmas have been described previously[1,2]

The chronic inflammation was described cytologically by the presence of clumps of hyperplastic mesothelial cells and a great number of lymphocytes and plasmocytes and histologically by fibrinoid exudates and areas of necrotic tissue surrounded by inflammatory cells.

A statistical analysis was made using the χ^2 test with Yates' correction for continuity.

RESULTS

The 74 patients were, in majority, of caucasian origin. They were 19–42 years old (mean 30.5 years, SD$\pm$4). Sixteen (21%) had a past history of salpingitis; seven (9%) had a past history of slight pelvic pain which could be interpreted as a subacute and non-treated salpingitis. Fifty-two (70%) had never had any sign of pelvic infection. None of them had any clinical or biological sign of inflammation at the time they requested treatment for sterility. Thirty-three (44%) had visible signs of chronic inflammation at laparoscopy; 46 (62%) had histological or cytological signs of chronic inflammation, 52 (70%) had either visible inflammation or only microscopical inflammation.

In the whole series, CT laparoscopic cultures were positive in 17 cases (23%), the IgG level was> 1/16 in 49 cases (66%) and> 1/128 in 16 cases (21%).

There is no significant difference between women with visible inflammation versus women without, for serodiagnosis. There is a significant difference for positive cultures (abdomen or cervix) ($p<0.01$).

There is a significant difference between women with histological or cytological inflammation for positive CT cultures ($p<0.001$), and IgG level > 1/128 ($p<0.003$). There is no significant difference for IgG> 1/16.

DISCUSSION

The results of this study confirm our previous works and those of Punnonen[3], showing a strong correlation between positive CT cultures, positive CT serology and sterilities due to tubal factors. This data was confirmed by that of Jones[4] and by animal experimentation carried out by Schachter[5].

In addition, the present study shows a strong correlation between CT evolutive infection and histological chronic inflammation, which was, a short time ago, described as giving no cultures for any bacteria and being auto-maintained[6]. The correlation with positive cultures is stronger if there is a histological inflammation than if there is a macroscopic inflammation.

References

1. Henry-Suchet, J., Catalan, F., Loffredo, V. *et al.* (1980). Microbiology of specimens obtained by laparoscopy from controls and from patients with pelvic inflammatory disease or infertility with tubal obstruction. *Am. J. Obst. Gynecol.*, **138**, 1022
2. Catalan, F., Khoury, B. and Siboulet, A. (1979). Diagnostic bacteriologiques des Chlamydia humaines. *Bull. Mem. Soc. Med. Paris.*, **7**, 60
3. Punnonen, R., Terho, P., Nikkanen, V. and Meurman, O. (1979). Chlamydia serology in infertile women by immunofluorescence. *Fertil. Steril.*, **31**, 656
4. Jones, R. B., Andery, B. R., Hui, S. L. and Cleary, R. E. (1982). Correlation between serum antichlamydial antibodies and tubal factor as a cause of infertility. *Fertil. Steril.*, **5**, 553
5. Schachter, J., Banks, J., Sung, M. and Sweet, R. (1982). Hydrosalpinx as a consequence of chlamydial salpingitis in the guinea pig. In P. A. Mardh, *et al.* (eds.) *Chlamydial Infections.* p. 371. (Amsterdam: Elsevier Biomedical Press)
6. De Brux, J. and Palmer, R. (1979). Nomenclature histologique des lesions inflammatoires tubaires. In *Oviducte et Fertilité.* p. 197. (Paris: Masson)

13
Specific IgG and IgA antibodies to *Chlamydia trachomatis* in infertile women

I. SAROV, D. KLEINMAN, R. CEVENINI, G. HOLCBERG, G. POTASHNIK, B. SAROV, N. KIMMEL and V. INSLER

INTRODUCTION

Recent studies have implicated *Chlamydia (C.) trachomatis* as one of the major causes of pelvic inflammatory disease (PID) which may lead to subsequent infertility[1-3]. Infertility could result from tubular damage due to chronic infection or as a result of acute salpingitis.

In this study we examined the prevalence of *C. trachomatis* IgG, IgA and IgM antibodies in infertile women and in matched controls by the single antigen (L-2) immunoperoxidase assay[4] recently developed in this laboratory.

MATERIALS AND METHODS

Human sera

Sera were obtained from four different groups. The control sera included:

(1) 50 sera from primiparous women obtained within 72 hours following delivery (mean age 23 years; range 20–26 years); (2) fifty sera from multiparous women (fourth delivery or more obtained in the 72 hours post partum (mean age 34 years; range 28–40 years). The infertile study population included 50 sera from women with unexplained infertility (mean age 29 years; range 24–42 years). The couples with unexplained infertility were defined as follows: infertility of at least 2 years' duration; normal pelvic findings;

evidence of ovulation (basal body temperature (BBT) and progesterone values); patent tubes (hysterosalpingography (HSG) and/or laparoscopy); normal prolactin levels and normal post-coital test (PCT) in the wife; no pathological findings in general physical and genital examinations; and normal seminal fluid analysis (SFA) in the husband; *in vitro* sperm penetration (SP) was normal in all couples. The last group comprised 30 sera from infertile women with abnormal HSG in one or both tubes (mean age 32; range 27–37 years).

Immunoperoxidase antibody assay (IPA)

The procedure is a modification of those described previously[4-6]. A dark blue cytoplasmic stain of *C. trachomatis* inclusion is easily recognized under the microscope. Known positive and negative sera were included in each assay. *C. trachomatis* IgG titres of over 4 or *C. trachomatis* IgA titres of over 2 were considered positive.

RESULTS

Table 1 demonstrates the distribution of chlamydial IgG and IgA antibody titres among 50 infertile women with normal HSG, 30 infertile women with abnormal HSG and 100 health controls.

C. trachomatis IgG antibodies – Infertile women with abnormal HSG showed significantly ($p<0.0001$) higher rates of *C. trachomatis* IgG seropositivity than control groups (87% *v.* 20% and 10% respectively, total $\chi^2=72.1$). A higher prevalence of *C. trachomatis* IgG antibodies was found also in infertile women with normal HSG than in control women (20% *v.* 10%). However, this difference was not found to be statistically significant ($p<0.20$). The GMT of the patients with mechanical sterility (20.7) was significantly higher than that of controls (5.6) ($p<0.01$). Relatively high *C. trachomatis* IgG titres (> 64) were observed in 27% of the abnormal HSG group and in 15% of the infertile women with normal HSG while none of the healthy controls had IgG titres of over 64.

C. trachomatis IgA antibodies – Infertile women with abnormal HSG showed significantly ($p<0.0001$) higher prevalence rates of IgA antibodies to *C. trachomatis* than control groups (77% *v.* 14% and 3% respectively, total $\chi^2=72.99$). A significantly ($p<0.05$) higher prevalence of *C. trachomatis* IgA antibodies was found in infertile patients with normal HSG in comparison with healthy control groups (14% *v.* 3%). The GMT of women with normal and abnormal HSG were higher than controls (19.3 and 13.2 *v.* 4.0 respectively). Relatively high *C. trachomatis* IgA titres (> 32) were observed in 43% of the abnormal HSG group versus 33% of infertile women with normal HSG

Table 1 Prevalence of IgG and IgA antibodies to *Chlamydia trachomatis* in infertile women *versus* comparison group

		IgG antibodies			*IgA antibodies*		
Study group	*No. tested*	*Percentage positive*	*GMT*	*Percentage with titre > 64*	*Percentage positive*	*GMT*	*Percentage with titre > 32*
Infertile women with abnormal HSG	30	87	20.7	27	77	13.2	33
Infertile women with normal HSG	50	20	10.5	10	14	19.3	43
Healthy women	100	10	5.6	0	3	4.0	0
Total	180	46			33		
Statistical significance (χ^2 test)		$p<0.0001$			$p<0.0001$		

HSG = Hysterosalpingogram.

while none of the control group had IgA titres of over 32.

C. trachomatis IgM antibodies – No *C. trachomatis* IgM antibodies (titre < 2) were found in any of the infertile or control group by the immunoperoxidase technique. Of the 30 patients with abnormal HSG only three had recalled having pelvic infections which indicates that most of these patients had asymptomatic PID.

DISCUSSION

C. trachomatis, a microbial obligate parasite, with a genome of about 670×10^6 daltons has become a major concern of modern medicine[7-9]. Recent investigations have been centred on the role of *C. trachomatis* in acute and chronic salpingitis which might lead to infertility. Salpingitis may be caused by a variety of organisms, the relative importance of which, however, seems to vary in different populations[1,10]. In a recent study, Mardh *et al.*[10], examining paired sera from 60 consecutive patients with acute salpingitis confirmed by laparoscopy, have obtained evidence from culture and/or serological tests that acute salpingitis in Lund, Sweden, is associated with a concurrent genital chlamydial infection in 58% of patients, whereas gonococcal infection and *Mycoplasma hominis* occur in 8% and 12%, respectively. Chlamydial antibody titres correlated with the severity of the tubal inflammation (as shown by laparoscopy) and the duration of the lower abdominal pains before attendance.

In the present study we have shown that infertile women have higher prevalence of and elevated IgG antibody titres to *C. trachomatis* than controls. The higher prevalence of *C. trachomatis* IgG antibody was significantly greater in infertile women with abnormal HSG as compared with infertile patients with normal HSG (87% *v.* 20%, respectively). These results are in agreement with those shown in different patient group studies in Europe and the United States[11-14] and support the hypothesis that *C. trachomatis* could be an important microbiological agent in tubal infertility. The fact that only 10% of the infertile women with abnormal HSG in the present study recalled having PID indicated that most of those infections were asymptomatic. Similar findings were observed also in other infertile groups[11,12,14] studied which suggest that subclinical *C. trachomatis* might be a major cause of tubal damage. Since no specific IgM was detected in our patients and the half-life of IgA is 5–6 days in normal persons[15] the presence of these antibodies might suggest continuous antigen stimulus due to chronic infection by *C. trachomatis*. The significantly higher prevalence of *C. trachomatis* IgA antibodies in infertile women with normal HSG versus controls (14% versus 3%) suggests that some of the women in this study might have a minor and probably initial stage of *C. trachomatis* infection in their fallopian tubes[16].

References

1. Westrom, L. and Mardh, P.A. (1982). Genital chlamydial infections in the female. In Mardh, P.A. *et al.* (eds.) *Chlamydial Infections.* pp. 121–139. (Amsterdam: Elsevier Biomedical Press)
2. Shachter, J. (1978). Chlamydia infections. *N. Engl. J. Med.*, **298**, 428–35, 490–95, 540–49
3. Sweet, R.L. (1982). Chlamydial salpingitis and infertility. *Fertil. Steril.*, **38**, 530
4. Cevenini, R., Rumpianesi, F., Donati, M. and Sarov, I. (1983). A rapid immunoperoxidase assay for the detection of specific IgG antibodies in *Chlamydia trachomatis. J. Clin. Pathol.*, **36**, 353
5. Haikin, H. and Sarov, I. (1980). Immunoperoxidase antibody to human cytomegalovirus-induced membrane antigen assay in the absence of interfering immunoglobulin G receptors. *Intervirology*, **14**, 155–9
6. Haikin, H. and Sarov, I. (1982). Determination of specific IgA antibodies to varicella zoster virus by immunoperoxidase assay. *J. Clin. Pathol.*, **35**, 645–9
7. Sarov, I. and Becker, Y. (1968). RNA in the elementary bodies of trachoma agent. *Nature (Lond.)*, **271**, 849
8. Sarov, I. and Becker, Y. (1969). Trachoma agent DNA. *J. Mol. Biol.*, **42**, 581–89
9. Moulder, J.W. (1982). A primer for chlamydiae. In Mardh, P.A. *et al.* (eds.) *Chlamydial Infections.* pp. 3–14. (Amsterdam: Elsevier Biomedical Press)
10. Mardh, P.A., Lind, I., Svensson, L., Westrom, l. and Moller, B.R. (1981). Antibodies to *Chlamydia trachomatis, Mycoplasma hominis* and *Neisseria gonorrhoeae* in sera from patients with acute salpingitis. *Br. J. Ven. Dis.*, **57**, 125–9
11. Punnonen, R., Terho, P., Nikkanen, V. and Meurman, O. (1979). Chlamydial serology in infertile women by immunofluorescence. *Fertil. Steril.*, **31**, 656–9
12. Gump, D.W., Gibson, M. and Ashikaga, T. (1982). Infertile women and *Chlamydia trachomatis* infection. In Mardh, P.A. *et al.* (eds.) *Chlamydial Infections.* pp. 193–6. (Amsterdam: Elsevier Biomedical Press)
13. Cevenini, R., Possati, G. and La Placa, M. (1982). *Chlamydia trachomatis* infection in infertile women. In Mardh, P.A., *et al.* (eds.) *Chlamydial Infections.* pp. 189–92. (Amsterdam: Elsevier Biomedical Press)
14. Jones, R.B., Ardery, B.R., Hui, S.L. and Cleary, R.E. (1982). Correlation between serum anti-chlamydial antibodies and tubal factor as a cause of infertility. *Fertil. Steril.*, **38**, 553
15. Tomasi, T.B. and Grey, H.M. (1972). Structure and function of immunoglobulin A. *Prog. Allergy*, **16**, 81–213
16. Sarov, I., Insler, V., Sarov, B., Cevenini, R., Rumpianesi, F., Donati, M., Kleinman, D., Piura, B., Lieberman, J., Kimmel, N., Friedman, M. and La Placa, M. (1984). Specific serum IgA antibodies in the diagnosis of active viral and chlamydial infections. *New Horizons in Microbiology.* (Elsevier Biomedical Press) (In press).

Acknowledgement

This work was supported in part by the Middle East Eye Research Institute (MEERI).

14
Tuberculosis of the female genital system

A. COMNINOS, E. TSAMANIS, T. LAINAS,
M. AL-ACHMAR and S. SARRIS

Tuberculosis of the female genital system is considered one of the main causes of infertility in Greece, although its incidence has dropped substantially during the last 40 years. The incidence of TB of the female genital system in Greece (Table 1) was reported as high as 2.5% between the years 1945 and 1953 but it dropped to 1% and 0.34% during the years 1953–1962 and 1962–1966, respectively.

Table 1 Incidence of TB of the female genital system

Investigator	*Years*	*Incidence (%)*
L. Kiriakis	1945–1953	2.5
J. Skliros	1953–1962	1.0
A. Comninos and E. Chryssikopoulos	1962–1966	0.34
A. Comninos *et al.*	1967–1976	0.64

In our present study which is based on the pathology reports of 6575 gynaecological operations performed in our hospital from 1967 to 1976 there were 42 cases of TB of the genital system which correspond to an incidence of 0.64%.

We would like to report here the preliminary results of a separate study which is still in progress. In a group of 28 cases selected at random among our infertility patients during the years 1978 to 1982 a sample of fluid was aspirated during laparoscopy from the pouch of Douglas and cultured for TB.

Furthermore, endometrial curretings taken from these patients during the first day of menstruation were also cultured for the same purpose. The age of these patients varied from 24 to 32 years and interestingly none of them mentioned a TB infection in the past and none of them complained of any symptoms besides sterility. Of the 28 cases the culture of the aspirated fluid from the pouch of Douglas was positive for TB in two (7%). These two patients also had positive cultures for TB from endometrial curretings.

Of the 42 cases of genital TB found between 6575 gynaecological operations, nine were post menopausal (48–61 years old) and 33 were in the reproductive period of life (21–44 years old). All 42 patients were married and 35 of them (83.3%) have never been pregnant. The remaining seven patients reported 1–3 pregnancies in the past (Table 2).

Table 2 Incidence of conception for 1967–1976 in women suffering TB of the female genital system

Conception	*No. of patients*	*Incidence (%)*
Never conceived	35	83.3
Conceived	7	16.7

The main reason for admission to hospital (Table 3) was in seven patients (16.6%) primary sterility, in one patient secondary infertility, in 22 patients (52.4%) menstrual disorders and in 10 patients (23.8%) abdominal pains. One patient was admitted for cancer of the cervix and one for relaxation of the pelvic floor.

Table 3 Main complaint on admission in patients with TB of the female genital system

Complaint	*1962–1966*	*1967–1976*	
	(%)	*No.*	*(%)*
Primary sterility	69.2	7	(16.6)
Secondary infertility	7.8	1	(2.4)
Menstrual disorders	30.0	22	(52.4)
Abdominal pain	22.4	10	(23.8)
Cervical cancer		1	(2.4)
Relaxation of pelvic floor		1	(2.4)

In our previous work for 1962–1966 there was a much higher percentage (69.2%) of primary sterility as the main reason for admission to hospital. However, although primary sterility is not mentioned as the main reason for admission in our present material, of 42 patients 83.3% of them have never conceived.

According to histological examination the TB infection of the genital system was located (Table 4) in the endometrium in 17 cases (40.5%), in both tubes in 10 cases (23.7%) and in one tube in six cases (14.3%). Furthermore, the TB infection was located in three cases in the endometrium and the endocervix, in two cases in the endometrium and one tube, in one case in the tube and the ovary, in one case in the endocervix and in one case in the omentum. Similar findings were found in our previous work of 1962–1968.

Table 4 Location of TB of the female genital system

Location	*1962–1966*	*1967–1976*	
	(%)	*No.*	*(%)*
Endometrium	38	17	(40.5)
One tube	19	6	(14.3)
Both tubes	26	10	(23.7)
Endometrium and one tube	17	2	(4.8)
Endometrium and both tubes		1	(2.4)
One tube and ovary		1	(2.4)
Endometrium and endocervix		3	(7.1)
Endocervix		1	(2.4)
Omentum		1	(2.4)

A previous extragenital TB infection (lungs, pleura, omentum) was reported as definite only in eight patients (19.0%) while another six patients mentioned a previous extragenital TB infection as possible. This gives a total of 14 cases (33.3%) with a previous definite and possible extragenital TB infection. It is worth noticing that all patients reported that the primary extragenital TB infection took place when they were young before the establishment of regular menstrual cycles.

In the material of 1962–1966 the percentage of extragenital TB infection was higher (42.3%). This difference is probably due to the improvement of the medical and sanitary conditions in our country as well as of the health services available which may restrict the classical manifestations of the primary TB infection and obscure the diagnosis.

Table 5 Findings of pelvic examination in patients with TB of the female genital system

	1962–1966	*1967–1976*	
	(%)	*No.*	*(%)*
Negative	65.3	29	(69.0)
Adnexal mass	34.7	2	(4.3)
Fibroids		9	(21.4)
Cervical cancer		1	(2.4)
Relaxation of pelvic floor		1	(2.4)

Besides the TB invasion of the genital system nine patients (21.4%) had fibroids of the uterus and one patient (3%) cancer of the cervix.

Also interesting are the findings of the pelvic examination (Table 5) performed on the day of admission to hospital. Examination was negative in 29 patients (69%), fibroids of the uterus were diagnosed in 21.4% and an adnexal mass was palpated in 4.8% of the patients. These findings correspond to the ones of our previous work.

From our study it can be concluded that:

(1) The frequency of TB of the female genital system in our country has dropped substantially from 2.5% to 0.4% between the years 1953 and 1966 and rose again slightly to 0.64% between the years 1967 and 1976.

(2) As the majority (83.3%) of our patients with TB of the genital system never conceived it can be assumed that TB of the female genital system constitutes a main cause of sterility.

(3) The female genital system is rather susceptible to TB infection. As the majority of the patients reported a primary extragenital TB infection before the establishment of menstruation it can be assumed that the susceptibility of the female genital system to TB is higher in teenagers, before the ripening of the endometrium and the tubal epithelium. The establishment of regular menstrual cycles and the ripening of the genital system apparently protects the endometrium and the tubes from the TB invasion. As far as the seven patients who reported 1–3 pregnancies in their history is concerned, the possibility that the TB infection of the genital system in these patients occurred after the birth of their children cannot be excluded.

(4) The majority of women (66.8%) with TB of the genital system did not mention in their past history an extragenital TB infection, and most of them were asymptomatic with a negative pelvic examination. Therefore it is advisable to include specific investigations for TB infection of the genital system in all cases of infertility and particularly in cases of primary sterility.

15
Resistant *Ureaplasma urealyticum* in infertile patients: a proposed method of treatment

H. W. HORNE, Jr. and R. B. KUNDSIN

In 1954, Maurice Shepard[1] first described T-stain mycoplasma (T for tiny) in the genitourinary tract of males with non-gonococcal urethritis ('non-specific urethritis') in his military population. Gnarpe and Friberg[2,3] and the present authors[4] in the early 1970s pioneered the concept of T-stain mycoplasma (now offically called *Ureaplasma urealyticum*, or UU) in association with human infertility and reproduction wastage. It was at this time that we first became aware of the already extensive appreciation by our veterinary colleagues of the role of mycoplasma infection in fertility problems in animals[5].

In the intervening decade, we first treated empirically using oral tetracycline without sensitivity testing. A number of treatment failures resulted. We then developed a method for sensitivity testing[6] and found that 13% of UU organisms cultured from infertile patients were resistant *in vitro* to tetracycline and its analogues at clinically safe levels.

We then tested the resistant strains with other antibiotics and various combinations of them and found that although *in vitro* some strains were susceptible in the laboratory, *in vivo* a clinical cure could not be attained. This left us with approximately 25 infertile couples who were incurable as far as their mycoplasma infection was concerned and who appeared after complete fertility work-up to have no other cause of their infertility.

Recently, Toth *et al.*[7] seem to have arrived at the same belief that mycoplasma can be an aetiological factor in human infertility. Also, Toth states that they have found a certain number of patients who are resistant to treatment and do not become pregnant. To our knowledge, Toth does not yet do sensitivity studies and thus is not aware of the resistant strains.

METHOD

In the summer of 1982, Dr Shepard suggested that we contact Dr Donald Griffith of the Department of Urology at Baylor University, whom he knew to be treating patients with staghorn renal calculi with aceto-hydroxamic acid (AHA)[8]. Dr Griffith believed that AHA was effective in suppressing urea splitting organisms like Proteus. Because there are reports in the literature that the nuclei of bladder calculi are often formed by ureaplasma colonies[9], it seemed reasonable to attempt *in vitro* sensitivity testing of AHA alone, and in combination with doxycycline and/or erythromycin. To our great surprise and pleasure, it worked *in vitro* against all resistant specimens tested when combined with both doxycycline and erythromycin, at clinically safe concentrations.

We therefore chose five infertile couples whose sensitivity tests showed totally resistant strains to all antibiotics and their combinations as candidates to whom the three medications would be administered simultaneously for 14 days, and who fully understood their problem and the nature of the experiment. Capsules of AHA were prepared containing 250 mg of the chemical and each couple (both husband and wife) self-administered one capsule four times daily along with 250 mg erythromycin four times daily. The Vibramycin 100 mg capsules were ordered by weight as is our usual advice (i.e. under 55 kg (120 lb), 1 capsule daily; 55–73 kg (120–160 lb), 1 capsule twice daily; 73–90 kg (160–200 lb), 1 capsule three times daily; and over 90 kg (200 lb), 1 capsule four times daily. All medication was begun on the second day of the wife's menstrual cycle for two reasons. First, we wanted to obtain the highest possible tissue drug levels and felt that with minimum endometrium present, this might improve results. Second, we wanted to stay away from the post-ovulatory phase as much as possible in case a pregnancy began.

Since these organisms are so sensitive that their re-growth is inhibited often for up to 2 months after receiving tetracycline medication, if a 100% lethal effect was not obtained, all patients had to wait for over 2 months after the end of treatment before being recultured. Normal coitus was allowed at all times in the hope of pregnancy.

RESULTS

Reculture was carried out only on the wife, as we find the organisms are more consistently found in the cervix, vagina, and female urethra than in the husband's genitourinary tract. Results have now been obtained in all five of the wives and all are negative.

DISCUSSION

A brief history of each couple is of interest to give a better perspective of the patients treated:

Couple 1.	Primary infertility (4 years).	
Couple 2.	Secondary infertility (1 year).	Had spontaneous abortion in 1981.
Couple 3.	Secondary infertility (2 years).	Had spontaneous abortion 1976, ectopic 1977. Had positive cultures, treated in 1978, normal baby 1980. Cultures resistant 1981 and 1982.
Couple 4.	Secondary infertility (2 years)	Had induced abortion 1973, spontaneous abortion 1980, same husband.
Couple 5.	Secondary infertility (1 year).	Wife had normal delivery in 1973, but the infant died ('cot death') in first marriage. Remarried 1979. Had reabsorbed pregnancies in 1979 and 1982.

Hence in this group of very infertile patients, there is only one living child resulting from nine pregnancies. We hope that clearing the chronic infection they all have had will help them attain normal families in the future. We shall now attempt to cure another larger group of 'resistant' patients and will report on our results as soon as possible. Parenthetically, it should be mentioned that there are those who suspect that mycoplasmas or ureaplasmas may play a part in the still unsolved syndrome of 'infant cot death' (see above).

Acknowledgements

This work was supported in part by the Reproduction Research Fund (Boston, Ma.) and the Kundsin Laboratory Inc. (Boston, Massachusetts). The authors would like to express their appreciation for the assistance given by Arthur T. Hertig, MD and Norval King, DVM of the Primate Center, Southboro, Massachusetts; by Sharon Poulin, microbiologist; by David Griffith, MD, Baylor Medical School, Houston, Texas; and by Paul Souney, BSR Ph, Brigham and Women's Hospital, Boston, Massachusetts.

References

1. Shepard, M. (1954). The recovery of pleuropneumonia-like organisms from Negro men with and without nongonococcal urethritis. *Am. J. Syph. Gon. Ven. Dis.*, **38**, 113
2. Gnarpe, H. and Friberg, J. (1972). Mycoplasma and human reproductive failure. *Am. J. Obstet. Gynecol.*, **114**, 727
3. Friberg, J. and Gnarpe, H. (1973). Mycoplasma and human reproductive failure. III – Pregnancies in 'infertile' couples treated with doxycycline for T-mycoplasma. *Am. J. Obstet. Gynecol.*, **116**, 23
4. Horne, H. W., Hertig, A. T., Kundsin, R. B. and Kosasa, T. S. (1973). Sub-clinical endometrial inflammation and T-mycoplasma: A possible cause of human reproductive failure. *Int. J. Fertil.*, **18**, 226
5. Gourlay, R. N. (1973). Significance of mycoplasma infection in cattle. *J. Am. Vet. Med. Assoc.*, **163**, 905
6. Spaepen, M. S. and Kundsin, R. B. (1977). Simple, direct broth-disk method for antibiotic susceptibility testing of *Ureaplasma urealyticum*. *Antimicrob. Agents Chemother.*, **11**, 267
7. Toth, A., *et al.* (1983). Subsequent pregnancies among 161 couples treated for T-mycoplasma genital-tract infection. *N. Engl. J. Med.*, **308**, 505
8. Griffith, D., Moskowitz, P. A. and Carlton, C. E., Jr. (1979). Adjunctive chemotherapy of infection-induced staghorn calculi. *J. Urol.*, **121**, 716
9. Friedlander, A. and Braude, A. (1974). production of bladder stones by human mycoplasma. *Nature (Lond.)*, **247**, 67

16
Prevalence of *Ureaplasma urealyticum* in habitual spontaneous abortion

W. FOULON, A. NAESSENS, M. VOLCKAERT and J. J. AMY

INTRODUCTION

The presence of ureaplasmas in the genital tract associated with spontaneous abortion was first reported by Kundsin *et al.* in 1967[1]. The possible association with fetal loss has since been investigated by several authors and frequently a positive correlation was found. Ureaplasmas were isolated more often from products of conception after first and mid-trimester abortion than those recovered after induced abortion[2,3]. However, it is not established from these studies whether the micro-organism is responsible for the fetal death or whether it only acts as a secondary invader of the already dead fetus. A prospective epidemiological survey was started to investigate the incidence of genital colonization with ureaplasmas in normal fertile patients and in patients with repeated pregnancy loss.

PATIENTS AND METHODS

Three groups of patients were studied. Group 1 comprised 34 normal fertile patients without previous spontaneous abortion; group 2, 104 patients having had one spontaneous abortion; and group 3, 31 patients with two or more spontaneous abortions. Cervical swabs were obtained in the three study groups; Stuart transport medium supplemented with charcoal was used. Endometrial specimens were obtained in groups 1 and 3. The endometrial sample was obtained with a narrow suction curette after disinfection of the cervix. Cultures were performed in bromothymol blue broth[4] and on differential agar medium A7[5].

RESULTS

U. urealyticum was found in the cervix in 15 out of 34 normal fertile women (44%), in 57 out of 104 women having had one spontaneous abortion (55%) and in 22 out of 31 patients (71%) with two or more spontaneous abortions. The difference in cervical isolation rate was statistically significant only in the group of patients with recurrent abortion ($p<0.05$).

Endometrium was positive for ureaplasmas in 12% of normal fertile women. Colonization rate was as high as 36% in patients with recurrent abortion ($p<0.05$) (Table 1).

Table 1 Presence of *Ureaplasma urealyticum* in the cervix and endometrium

Group	*Isolation from cervix*	*Isolation from endometrium*
Normal fertile woman ($n=34$)	15 (44%)	4 (12%)
One spontaneous abortion ($n=104$)	57 (55%)	
Recurrent abortion ($n=31$)	22 (71%)	11 (36%)*

* Results significantly different from normal ($p<0.05$)

However, considering only the patients with positive cervical cultures no significance was obtained ($p<0.25$) (Table 2). This is probably due to the small number of patients with positive cervical cultures studied.

Table 2 Presence of *Ureaplasma urealyticum* in endometrium in patients with positive cervical cultures

Group	*No. in group*	*No. with positive endometrial tissue*
Fertile population	15	4
Recurrent abortion	22	11

DISCUSSION

Considering the higher isolation rate of *U. urealyticum* in cervix and endometrium in patients with recurrent spontaneous abortions (71% and 36%, respectively) as compared with a control group of normal multigravidae (44% and 12%, respectively), the association between a maternal infection with *U. urealyticum* and spontaneous abortion is more than a simple coincidence. Our results confirm those of Stray-Pedersen *et al.*[6] who isolated more often the micro-organism from the endometrium in women who had recurrent spontaneous abortion (28%) than from a control group (7%). These findings suggest an association between a subclinical inflammation of the endometrium and spontaneous abortion. The low pathogenicity of this micro-organism is probably the reason for the absence of clinical signs of endometritis.

Nevertheless, numerous problems remain unsolved. Indeed an important percentage of normal pregnant women without a history of spontaneous abortion are colonized by the micro-organism. To determine why some women will abort and others will not, studies are necessary including serological investigation and serotyping of the different ureaplasma strains.

References

1. Kundsin, R. B., Driscoll, S. G. and Ming, P. L. (1967). Strain of mycoplasma associated with human reproductive failure. *Science*, **157**, 1573–4
2. Caspi, E., Solomon, F. and Sompolinsky, D. (1972). Early abortion and mycoplasma infection. *Isr. J. Med. Sci.*, **8**, 122–7
3. Sompolinsky, D., Solomon, F., Elkina, L., Weinraub, Z., Bukovsky, I. and Caspi, E. (1975). Infections with mycoplasmas and bacteria in induced mid-trimester abortion and fetal loss. *Am. J. Obstet. Gynecol.*, **121**, 610–16
4. Robertson, J. A. (1978). Bromothymol blue broth: Improved medium for detection of *Ureaplasma urealyticum* (T-strain mycoplasma). *J. Clin. Microbiol.*, **7**, 127–32
5. Shepard, M. C. and Lunceford, C. D. (1976). Differential agar medium (A7) for identification of *Ureaplasma urealyticum* (human T mycoplasmas) in primary cultures of clinical material. *J. Clin. Microbiol.*, **3**, 613–25
6. Stray-Pedersen, B. (1979). Female colonization with *Ureaplasma urealyticum* and reproductive failure. *Curr. Ther. Res.*, **26**, 771–8

Part III

Endometriosis

Part III

Section 1
Pathophysiology

17
Aetiology of infertility in patients with endometriosis

S. Z. A. BADAWAY, M. NUSBAUM, L. MARSHALL, V. CUENCA and R. CITTADINO

It is estimated that about 6–15% of infertile women have endometriosis. The aetiololgy of infertility in these patients is variable. Pelvic adhesions may lead to mechanical dysfunction in ovum pick-up phenomenon in severe endometriosis. However, infertility in mild and moderate endometriosis may be multifactorial and is still subject for research. It has been suggested that ovulatory dysfunction[1] and peritoneal fluid prostaglandins[2] are contributory factors to infertility in endometriosis patients. The present study attempts to evaluate these two aspects.

The incidence of ovulatory dysfunction was found to be 28% in 103 patients with endometriosis (5% anovulatory, 11% oligo-ovulatory, and 12% luteal phase inadequacy). There was no effect of duration of infertility, stage of endometriosis, or prior use of oral contraceptives on the ovulatory pattern. The mean age of patients with ovulatory dysfunction was significantly higher than patients with normal ovulatory cycles (30 ± 4.01 *v.* 27.8 ± 4.05 years, $p < 0.02$). Ovulatory dysfunction may be a function of age in patients with endometriosis, since no endocrinopathies were detected. Other investigators found ovulatory dysfunction in 16–79% of patients with endometriosis. Thus ovulatory dysfunction in patients with endometriosis is an important factor that should be corrected to increase the chances of achieving a pregnancy.

The concentration of prostaglandins $F_{2\alpha}$ and E_2 were evaluated in the peritoneal fluid of 38 patients with endometriosis and 35 control patients. Prostaglandin E_2 was significantly higher in endometriosis patients than controls during days 1–15 of the cycle (19.5±5.94 *v.* 8.62±2.86 ng ml^{-1}, $p<0.001$). On the other hand, there was significantly higher concentration of prostaglandin $F_{2\alpha}$ in endometriosis patients as compared with controls during days 16–28 of the cycle (2.78±1.42 *v.* (1.46±67 ng ml^{-1}, $p<0.025$).

Ovulatory dysfunction is an associated phenomenon in patients with endometriosis. The incidence in the present study is 28%, which is not different from observations by other investigators. It is also within the range of 10–40% seen in infertile women in general. This might suggest that endometriosis does not increase the incidence of ovulatory dysfunction. Nevertheless, it is essential to diagnose such dysfunction which seems to be more in the elderly group of patients. This might be due to hypothalamic pituitary ovarian dysfunction. Furthermore, excess prostaglandin concentrations in the peritoneal fluid in such patients might be an important additional contributory factor. Prostaglandin $F_{2\alpha}$, in high concentration, has been shown to inferfere with folliculogenesis and corpus luteum function in mice[3]. It is also luteolytic in humans and subhuman primates. In addition, experimentally induced endometriosis in rabbits leads to increased peritoneal fluid prostaglandins. It was suggested that the infertility in such rabbits was caused by anovulation[4].

Peritoneal fluid prostaglandins also might lead to dysfunction in tubal motility since prostaglandin $F_{2\alpha}$ is stimulatory and E_2 in inhibitory. Furthermore, high concentrations of both prostaglandins might inhibit the ciliary function of tubal endosalpinx. All of these factors interfere with proper ovum transfer phenomenon in the fallopian tube and thus will cause infertility[5,6].

References

1. Soules, M. R., Malinak, L. R., Bury, R. and Poindexter, A. (1976). Endometriosis and anovulation: A coexisting problem in the infertile female. *Am. J. Obstet. Gynecol.*, **125**, 412
2. Badawy, S. Z. A., Marshall, L., Gabal, A. A. and Nusbaum, M. L. (1982). The concentration of 13, 14-dihydro-15-keto prostaglandin $F_{2\alpha}$ and prostaglandin E_2 in peritoneal fluid of infertile patients with and without endometriosis. *Fertil. Steril.*, **38**, 166
3. Peluso, J. J., Leiper, S. and Steger, R. W. (1980). Effects of $PGF_{2\alpha}$ induced luteolysis and progesterone on follicular growth in pregnant mice. *Prostaglandins*, **19**, 437
4. Schenken, R. S. and Asch, R. H. (1980). Surgical induction of endometriosis in the rabbit: effect on fertility and concentrations of peritoneal fluid prostaglandins. *Fertil. Steril.*, **34**, 581
5. Barbosa, I. C., Maia, H., Jr., Durado, V. and Coutinho, E. M. (1980). Effect of prostaglandin $F_{2\alpha}$ on oviduct contractility in Marmoset monkeys. *Fertil. Steril.*, **33**, 197
6. Verdugo, P., Rumery, R. and Tarn, P. Y. (1980). Hormonal control of oviductal ciliary activity: effects of prostaglandins. *Fertil. Steril.*, **33**, 193

18
Peritoneal fluid 6-keto prostaglandin $F_{1\alpha}$ levels in women with endometriosis

T. J. MUDGE, W. R. JONES, J. A. WALSH and M. J. JAMES

INTRODUCTION

There is considerable evidence to support an association between endometriosis and infertility[1]. When the endometriosis is extensive and there is anatomical disorganization of the pelvis, such an association would seem to be readily explained on the basis of impaired ovum pick-up. With lesser degrees of endometriosis such an association, if indeed one exists, is much more difficult to explain.

It has been suggested that prostaglandins produced by the ectopic endometrium may interfere with ovarian function[2,3]. Prostaglandins are synthesized by endometrium[4] and it has been demonstrated that high concentrations of $PGF_{2\alpha}$ inhibit follicular growth in mice[5] and cause luteolysis in humans[6] and monkeys[7]. Furthermore, prostaglandins and thromboxane A_2 act on smooth muscle. If prostanoids are present in increased amounts in the peritoneum of women with endometriosis they might therefore affect tubal function. Studies addressing this possibility have shown inconsistent results. It has been reported that the levels of PGE_2, $PGF_{2\alpha}$, 15-keto-13-14-dihydro $PGF_{2\alpha}$ and thromboxane B_2 (TXB_2) are not elevated in the peritoneal fluid of women with endometriosis[8]. Conversely, it has been reported that levels of TXB_2 (the stable metabolite of TXA_2) and 6-keto $PGF_{1\alpha}$ (the stable metabolite of prostacyclin) are elevated in the peritoneal fluid of women with endometriosis[3].

In an attempt to resolve this issue, we have measured the concentration and determined the total amounts of 6-keto $PGF_{1\alpha}$ in the peritoneal fluid of 113 women who presented with infertility and who underwent laparoscopy as part of their investigation for this problem.

METHODS

Subjects

Women undergoing laparoscopy during the luteal phase of their menstrual cycle were studied. All women belonged to infertile couples but in some the cause of the infertility was a male factor. At laparoscopy, the total amount of peritoneal fluid lying free in the pouch of Douglas or in the utero-vesical pouch was aspirated into a syringe using a Verres needle through a second puncture. The diagnosis of endometriosis was made on the typical appearance of this condition, occasionally supplemented by biopsy and histological confirmation The control group included women with adhesions from old pelvic inflammatory disease or surgery, fallopian tube occlusion and those where the pelvis was normal. No woman in this study was having hormone treatment. The peritoneal fluid was stored frozen until subsequent assay of prostaglandin levels.

Prostaglandin assays

Aliquots (0.5 ml) of peritoneal fluid were acidified (1 $moll^{-1}$ HCl, 100 μl) and $_3H$-labelled 6-keto $PGF_{1\alpha}$ (0.005 μCi) was added. Prostaglandins were extracted with ethyl acetate. This solvent was evaporated with nitrogen and 0.5 ml Na_2CO_3 (100 $\mu moll^{-1}$, pH 10) were added to the residue. Aliquots (0.1 ml) of this solution were used to calculate the extraction efficiency and to estimate the amount of 6-keto $PGF_{1\alpha}$ by radioimmunoassay (RIA). The RIA system employed commercially available antisera (Seragen Inc., Boston), ^3H-labelled 6-keto $PGF_{1\alpha}$ (Amersham International, Sydney), and 6-keto $PGF_{1\alpha}$ (Cayman Chemical, Denver). Determinations were usually performed in triplicate unless under 1.5 ml of peritoneal fluid was collected.

RESULTS

Peritoneal fluid concentrations of 6-keto $PGF_{1\alpha}$ and the volumes of collected peritoneal fluid were measured in 113 women. Of this group, 42 women had evidence of endometriosis at laparoscopy and 71 women had no evidence of this disease. The concentrations of 6-keto $PGF_{1\alpha}$ in the two groups are represented in Figure 1. The median values for the two groups are similar (Table 1) although the larger median value is only $3.2\,ng\,ml^{-1}$, the overall range is very large, extending from 0.8 to $98.2\,ng\,ml^{-1}$. The values for the two groups were compared by using the Mann–Whitney U test (two-tailed) and no difference between the two groups was found ($\alpha=0.05$).

Because prostaglandin concentration is a function of the volume of fluid and the total amount of prostaglandin present, we have also recorded these individual parameters. The distributions of peritoneal fluid volumes appear

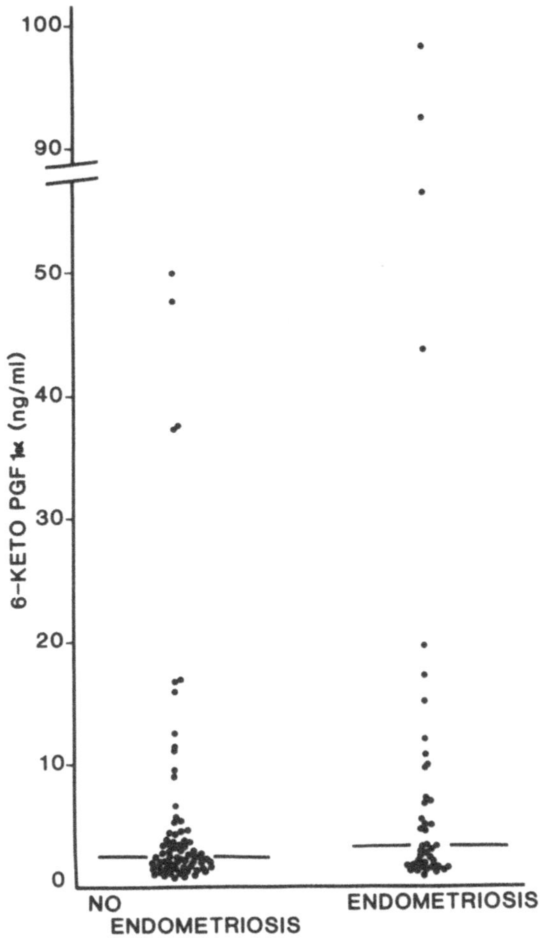

Figure 1 Peritoneal fluid concentration of 6-keto $PGF_{1\alpha}$. Horizontal lines indicate the median values

Table 1 Median values of peritoneal fluid volumes and levels of 6-keto $PGF_{1\alpha}$

Group	*6-keto $PGF_{1\alpha}$ concentrations* (ng ml^{-1})	*6-keto $PGF_{1\alpha}$ total amount* (ng)	*Volume* (ml)
Endometriosis (n=42)	3.2	24.9	9.1
Non-endometriosis (n=71)	2.4	25.1	9.0

similar in the two groups (Figure 2) and the median values of the two groups are similar (Table 1). When the peritoneal fluid volumes of the two clinical groups were compared (Mann–Whitney U test), no difference was found (α=0.05, two-tailed). The median values for the total amount of 6-keto $PGF_{1\alpha}$ present in peritoneal fluid were similar for the two groups (Table 1) and although the median values were approximately 25 ng the combined range of

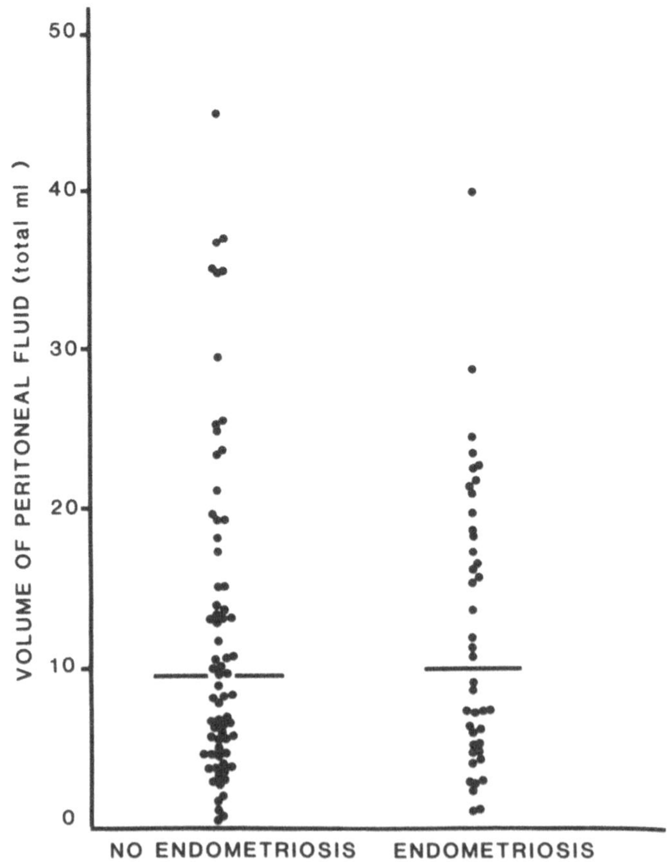

Figure 2 Peritoneal fluid volumes. Horizontal lines indicate the median values

values extended from 1 to 996 ng (Figure 3). There was no difference in total prostaglandin levels between the two groups when compared by the Mann–Whitney U test ($\alpha=0.05$, two-tailed).

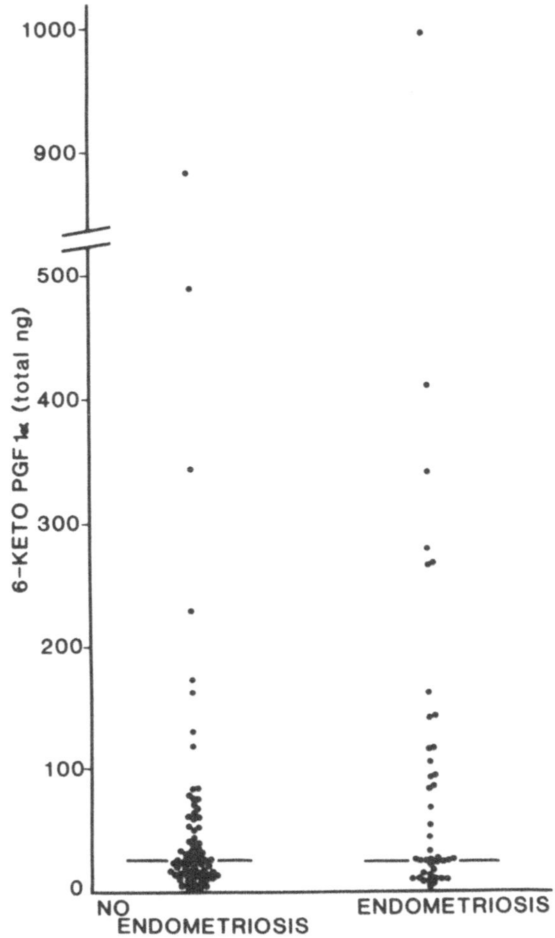

Figure 3 Total amounts of peritoneal fluid 6-keto $PGF_{1\alpha}$. Horizontal lines indicate the median values

DISCUSSION

The results of our study indicate that neither the amount nor the concentration of 6-keto $PGF_{1\alpha}$ in peritoneal fluid of women with endometriosis was different from that in women with no macroscopic evidence of endometriosis. These results conflict with those reported by Drake *et al.*[3] who found that both the amount and concentration of TXB_2 and 6-keto $PGF_{1\alpha}$ were increased in the peritoneal fluid of women with endometriosis ($n=14$) when compared with women without endometriosis ($n=15$). However, the conclusions of Drake *et al.*[3] must be considered equivocal due to several aspects of their study methodology. Firstly, the authors do not indicate if all peritoneal fluid was sampled at either pre- or post-ovulatory time points, and secondly they exclude from their non-endometriosis group three women with unexplained infertility who had high levels of 6-keto $PGF_{1\alpha}$ and TXB_2 similar to those in their endometriosis group. Although the authors suggest that microscopic endometriosis may have been present in these three women, if this was not visible macroscopically it seems invalid to exclude them. A further problem with the data is the inappropriate use of the *t*-test to analyse data that is not normally distributed[9].

Although Rock *et al.*[8] did not measure 6-keto $PGF_{1\alpha}$, they reported that the peritoneal fluid concentrations of PGE_2, $PGF_{2\alpha}$, PGFM and TXB_2 in women with endometriosis were not different from the concentrations in women with no evidence of endometriosis. The results of Rock *et al.*[8] parallel our results with 6-keto $PGF_{1\alpha}$ levels although these investigators sampled peritoneal fluid during the proliferative phase of the menstrual cycles whereas we sampled fluid during the luteal phase for this study. In agreement with Rock *et al.*[8], we have found no difference in peritoneal fluid volumes between these two groups of women. In contrast, Drake *et al.*[10] reported that the peritoneal fluid volumes of women with endometriosis were greater than those of women without endometriosis throughout the menstrual cycle.

Comparisons of these studies under discussion are difficult for several reasons. The time points of the menstrual cycle at which peritoneal fluid was sampled were either not reported or were different for each study. Furthermore, the non-endometriosis groups of these studies are variously comprised of presumably fertile women undergoing elective sterilization, infertile women with pelvic disorders and women with unexplained infertility with no evidence of a pelvic factor.

It would be difficult to find a control group in whom this possibility could be excluded. We have measured 6-keto $PGF_{1\alpha}$ in a small control group of ten patients undergoing laparoscopic sterilization in the luteal phase in their cycle. They were either not contracepting or using barrier methods. There was no significant difference in concentration or total amounts of 6-keto $PGF_{1\alpha}$ between this control group and those with endometriosis reported above.

In no single study have all of the principal prostanoids (PGE_2, $PGF_{2\alpha}$, 6-keto $PGF_{1\alpha}$, TXB_2) been measured. But it is apparent that all of these prostanoids are present in various amounts in peritoneal fluid and it is probable that they arise from various sources. Prostaglandin F is produced by human follicles[11],

PGE and PGF are produced by human corpora lutea[12], PGE_2 and $PGF_{2\alpha}$ are produced by human endometrial stroma cells[4] and 6-keto $PGF_{1\alpha}$ and PGE_2 are formed by rabbit mesothelial cells[13]. 6-keto $PGF_{1\alpha}$ was not synthesized by human endometrium in one study[14]. We are not aware of attempts to detect 6-keto $PGF_{1\alpha}$ synthesis by human follicles or corpora lutea. The source of human peritoneal fluid 6-keto $PGF_{1\alpha}$ may be the mesothelial cells of the peritoneum or it may prove to be the ovaries. Whatever the source, peritoneal fluid 6-keto $PGF_{1\alpha}$ levels were not elevated in women with endometriosis in this study.

ACKNOWLEDGEMENTS

We wish to thank Miss L. Thorpe for expert technical assistance.

References

1. Strathy, J. H., Molgaard, C. A., Coulam, C. B. and Melton, L. J. (1982). Endometriosis and infertility: a laparoscopic study of endometriosis among fertile and infertile women. *Fertil. Steril.*, **38**, 667
2. Schenken, R. S. and Asch, R. H. (1980). Surgical induction of endometriosis in the rabbit: effects on fertility and concentrations of peritoneal fluid prostaglandins. *Fertil. Steril.*, **34**, 581
3. Drake, T. S., O'Brien, W. F., Ramwell, P. W. and Metz, S. A. (1981). Peritoneal fluid thromboxane B_2 and 6-keto $PGF_{1\alpha}$ in endometriosis. *Am. J. Obstet. Gynecol.*, **140**, 401
4. Gal, D., Casey, M. L., Johnston, J. M. and MacDonald, P. C. (1982). Mesenchyme-epithelial interactions in human endometrium. Prostaglandin synthesis in separated cell types. *J. Clin. Invest.*, **70**, 798
5. Peluso, J. J., Leiper, S. and Steger, R. W. (1980). Effects of $PGF_{2\alpha}$ induced luteolysis and progesterone on follicular growth in pregnant mice. *Prostaglandins*, **19**, 437
6. Wentz, A. C. and Jones, G. S. (1973). Transient luteolytic effect of prostaglandin $F_{2\alpha}$ in the human. *Obstet. Gynaecol.*, **42**, 172
7. Shaikh, A. (1972). Luteal regression in monkeys after the administration of estradiol and prostaglandin $F_{2\alpha}$. *Prostaglandins*, **2**, 227
8. Rock, J. A., Dubin, N. H., Ghodgaonkar, R. B., Bergquist, C. A., Erozan, Y. S. and Kimball, A. W. (1982). Cul-de-sac fluid in women with endometriosis: fluid volume and prostanoid concentration during the proliferative phase of the cycle – days 8 to 12. *Fertil. Steril.*, **37**, 747
9. Hall, J. C. (1982). Use of the t-test in the *British Journal of Surgery*. *Br. J. Surg.*, **69**, 55
10. Drake, T., O'Brien, W., Grunert, G. and Metz, S. (1980). Peritoneal fluid volumes in endometriosis. *Fertil. Steril.*, **34**, 280
11. Armstrong, D. (1981). Prostaglandins and follicular functions. *J. Reprod. Fertil.*, **62**, 283
12. Patwardhan, V. V. and Lanthier, A. (1980). Concentration of prostaglandins PGE and PGF, esterone, estradiol and progesterone in human corpora lutea. *Prostaglandins*, **20**, 963
13. Coene, M. C., Van Hove, C., Claeys, M. and Herman, A. G. (1982). Arachidonic acid metabolism by cultured mesothelial cells. *Biochim. Biophys. Acta*, **710**, 437
14. Green, K., Christensen, N. and Bygdeman, M. (1981). The chemistry and pharmacology of prostaglandins, with reference to human reproduction. *J. Reprod. Fertil.*, **62**, 269

19

Decreased concentration of ovarian LH(hCG) receptor in polycystic ovarian disease and endometriosis

A. KAUPPILA, H. RAJANIEMI and L. RÖNNBERG

INTRODUCTION

Undisturbed LH action is essential for normal follicular maturation, ovulation and corpus luteum formation. In polycystic ovarian disease (PCOD), pituitary LH secretion, at least in relation to FSH secretion, is pathologically high[1]. There are also diseases, e.g. endometriosis[2], known often to be accompanied by unexplained infertility in spite of apparently normal concentrations of circulating gonadotrophins. In such conditions the follicular membrane receptors mediating the action of LH might be at fault. For these reasons we measured the LH(hcG) receptor concentrations of the Graafian follicle or the corpus luteum cells of patients suffering from PCOD or endometriosis.

MATERIALS AND METHODS

Twelve patients with PCOD, 51 patients with endometriosis and 41 control subjects with no infertility problems or ovarian affections were selected for this study. At operation ovarian wedge resection was performed. The tissue specimen was immediately frozen and stored at −60 °C until assayed for LH(hCG) receptor. In endometriosis and control cases the granulosa cells of the largest ovarian follicle, or fresh corpus luteum, and in PCOD, cell samples from the cystic follicles, were taken for LH(hCG) determination using

[^{125}I]iodo-hCG as a ligand hormone. A detailed description of the method has been given elsewhere[3].

RESULTS

The ovarian follicles of patients with PCOD or endometriosis had significantly lower concentrations of LH(hCG) receptors than those of the control subjects (Figure 1, Table 1). In addition, three of 12 specimens from PCOD patients, and six out of 36 specimens from endometriosis patients did not show specific binding of [^{125}I]iodo-hCG.

In endometriosis the LH(hCG) receptor concentration remained constant throughout the follicular phase of the menstrual cycle, while in the control

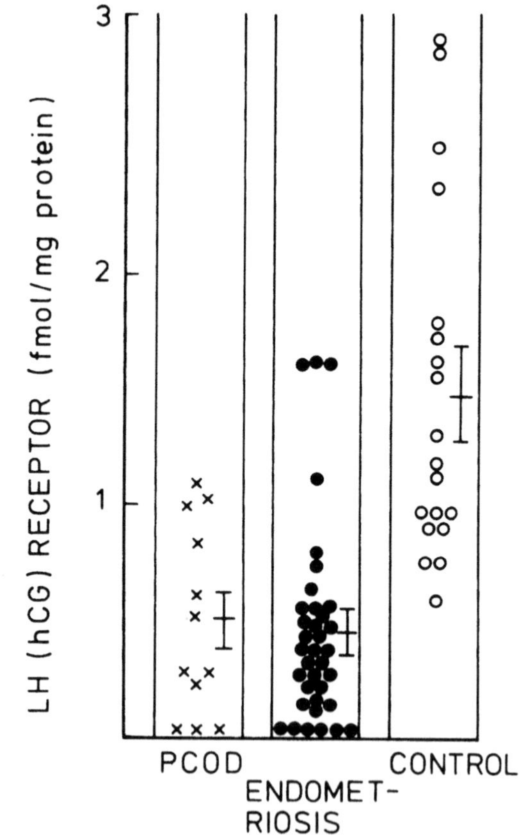

Figure 1 Individual and mean ± SE concentrations of LH(hCG) receptors in normal ovarian follicles and in those of patients with polycystic disease (PCOD) or endometriosis

Table 1 Mean (±SE) LH(hCG) receptor concentrations in ovarian follicles and corpora lutea of patients with endometriosis and control subjects without endometriosis or other ovarian affections at different phases of the menstrual cycle

Cycle days	*No. of patients*	*Endometriosis LH(hCG) receptors* (fmol (mg homogenate protein)$^{-1}$)	*No. of controls*	*Controls LH(hCG) receptors* (fmol (mg homogenate protein)$^{-1}$)	*Significance of difference*
6–10	19	0.43±0.11	8	1.31±0.27	$p<0.001$
11–15	17	0.48±0.10	11	1.59±0.22	$p<0.001$
14–19	8	3.92±0.72	11	3.58±0.77	NS
20–30	7	2.62±0.55	11	4.62±0.65	$p<0.05$

NS=not significant.

patients the receptor concentration increased (Table 1). In severe and extensive endometriosis the mean ($\pm$SE) LH(hCG) receptor concentration (0.28 ± 0.07 fmol (mg homogenate protein)$^{-1}$) was lower ($p < 0.05$) than in mild or moderate disease (0.61 ± 0.21 fmol (mg homogenate protein)$^{-1}$). During the late but not the early luteal phase of the cycle the LH(hCG) receptor concentration of the corpus luteum was significantly decreased in cases of endometriosis (Table 1).

DISCUSSION

In this study we have summarized our previous observations of [^{125}I]iodo-hCG binding to the ovaries of the patients with PCOD[3] or endometriosis[4,5]. Our results showed that the ovarian follicles of patients with PCOD or endometriosis contained receptors for luteinizing hormone. However, in relation to normally developing follicles, the number of LH(hCG) receptors was significantly decreased. For this reason, the sensitivity of the granulosa cells to LH stimulation might be diminished and ovulation and the development of the corpus luteum disturbed.

In cases of PCOD the tonic elevation of serum LH concentrations, typical of this disease[1], may cause down-regulation of LH(hCG) receptors, and lead to a derangement in follicular maturation[3,6]. In a rat model for PCOD, Copman and Adams[7] also observed low concentrations of LH(hCG) receptors and high numbers of FSH receptors in cystic follicles.

In cases of endometriosis the serum concentrations of gonadotrophins do not deviate from normal to such an extent that might explain the low concentration of follicular LH(hCG) receptors. Muse and co-workers[8] recently observed that the prolactin response to TRH stimulus was increased in endometriosis, possibly suggesting relative hyperprolactinaemia. This finding is interesting because hyperprolactinaemia disturbs folliculogenesis in patients with pituitary prolactinoma[9] and in experimental conditions[10]. Further studies, however, are needed to explore the significance of prolactin in endometriosis and in the development of the ovarian follicle.

References

1. Spellacy, W. N. (1981). Polycystic ovarian disease. *Fertil. Steril.*, **36**, 306
2. Dmowski, W. P. (1981). Current concepts in the management of endometriosis. *Obstet. Gynecol. Ann.*, **10**, 279
3. Rajaniemi, H., Rönnberg, L., Kauppila, A., Ylöstalo, P. and Vihko, R. (1980). Luteinizing hormone receptors in ovarian follicles of patients with polycystic ovarian disease. *J. Clin. Endocrinol. Metab.*, **51**, 1054
4. Kauppila, A., Rajaniemi, H. and Rönnberg, L. (1982), Low LH(hCG) receptor concentration in ovarian follicles in endometriosis. *Acta Obstet. Gynecol. Scand.*, **61**, 81

5. Rönnberg, L., Kauppila, A. and Rajaniemi, H. (1984). LH(hCG) receptor disorder in endometriosis. *Fertil. Steril.* (In press)
6. Rao, Ch.V. (1982). Receptors for gonadotropins in human ovaries. In *Recent Advances in Fertility Research*. Part A: *Developments in Reproductive Endocrinology*. pp. 123–35. (New York: Alan R. Liss)
7. Copman, T.L. and Adams, W.C. (1981). Ovarian gonadotropin receptor during experimental ovarian cyst formation in the rat. *Biol. Reprod.*, **25**, 115
8. Muse, K., Wilson, E.A. and Jawad, M.J. (1982). Prolactin hyperstimulation in response to thyrotropin-releasing hormone in patients with endometriosis. *Fertil. Steril.*, **38**, 542
9. McNeilly, A.S. (1980). Paradoxical prolactin. *Nature (Lond.)*, **284**, 212
10. Kauppila, A., Leinonen, P., Vihko, R. and Ylöstalo, P. (1982). Metoclopramide-induced hyperprolactinaemia impairs ovarian follicle maturation and corpus luteum formation in women. *J. Clin. Endocrinol. Metab.*, **54**, 955

20
Autoimmune phenomena in infertile patients with endometriosis

S. Z. A. BADAWY, V. CUENCA, A. STITZEL,
R. D. B. JACOBS and R. H. TOMAR

Recent data in the literature suggest that endometriosis may lead to an autoimmune reaction. This is supported by the presence of excess macrophage reaction in the peritoneal fluid of these patients[1]. In addition, immunofluorescence studies have shown the presence of complement component C3 in the endometrium of patients with endometriosis[2]. It has been hypothesized that protein substances from the ectopic endometrial tissue is recognized as foreign and stimulate the immune reaction. The present study examines the concentration of complement components C3c and C4, properdin, factor B, and immunoglobulins in the peritoneal fluid and serum of infertile patients with endometriosis. The results are compared with those with no evidence of endometriosis.

The concentration of C3c and C4 is significantly increased in serum and peritoneal fluid of patients with endometriosis compared with controls ($p < 0.01$) (Table 1). There was no significant difference in the concentration of properdin and factor B between endometriosis and control patients. In addition, there was no significant difference in the concentration of immunoglobulins G, A and M between endometriosis and control patients.

The complement system is an amplifier of the immune response in the body. This may be through the classical or the alternative pathways. The classical pathway is activated by immunoglobulins G and M and C-reactive protein. The alternative pathway is activated by immunoglobulins A and G and bacterial polysaccharides[3]. The results of the present study show increased

Table 1 Mean (±SD) Concentration of complement component C3c and C4 in serum and peritoneal fluid*

	Control		*Endometriosis*	
Serum (mg dl^{-1})				
C3c	55.16±13.40	(27)	67.08±17.09	(26)†
C4	19.11± 6.27	(25)	28.14±11.34	(25)†
Peritoneal fluid (mg dl^{-1})				
C3c	31.73±11.06	(27)	42.99±14.63	(26)†
C4	9.68±2.05	(25)	17.18± 9.42	(25)†

* Number of patients given in parentheses.
† Difference between control and endometriosis groups significant ($p<0.05$).

complement component C3c and C4 in peritoneal fluid and serum of endometriosis reactions. The increase of the complement components in the peritoneal fluid suggests an antigen–antibody reaction in the peritoneal cavity of these patients. The increase of the complement components in the serum may represent an increased turnover that suggests an increased synthesis. The lack of increase in factor B and properdin in endometriosis patients might suggest that the putative immune reaction leads to activation of complement system by the classical pathway.

Further studies are in progress in our laboratories to identify the nature of the antigen and any precipitation reactions with the serum or peritoneal fluid of patients with endometriosis.

References

1. Haney, A. F., Muscato, J. J. and Weinberg, J. B. (1981). Peritoneal fluid cell populations in infertility patients. *Fertil. Steril.*, **35**, 696
2. Weed, J. C. and Arquembroug, P. C. (1980). Endometriosis: Can it produce an autoimmune response resulting in infertility? *Clin. Obstet. Gynecol.*, **23**, 885
3. Cooper, N. R. (1980). The complement system. In Fundenberg, H. H., Stites, D. P., Caldwell, J. L. and Wells, J. V. (eds.) *Basic and Clinical Immunology*. 3rd Edn. pp. 83–95. (Los Altos, Ca.: Lange Medical Publications)

Part III

Section 2
Therapy and Results

21
Endoscopic cytopuncture in the diagnosis of intraovarian endometriosis

M. MINTZ and J. DE BRUX

During 4066 laparoscopies performed over 21 years among unselected patients, 468 explorative cytopunctures were performed. These punctures contributed to the endoscopic screening of endometriosis by including every ovarian cyst or suspected intraovarian lesion which appeared neither as a growing follicle nor a vascularized corpus luteum. The complete results were as follows:

(1) 54 dermoid cysts.
(2) 116 seromucoid cysts.
(3) 298 haematic cysts or intraovarian deposits:
    (a) 150 persistent folliculoluteinic cysts;
    (b) 148 cases of intraovarian endometriosis;
        (i) 75 cysts surrounded by endometriotic signs;
        (ii) 73 ovaries without endometriotic signs (31 ordinary looking cysts and 42 invisible intraovarian deposits).

These results showed the two advantages of cytopuncture:

(1) The elimination of 150 haematic luteal cysts which could easily be confused with endometriosis in the absence of cytology.
(2) The surprising number of 73 cases of hidden intraovarian endometriosis without any visible stigmata, which would have escaped diagnosis if cytopuncture had not been done.

The reliability of cytology in endoscopic punctures is 86% as confirmed by 83 histopathological surgical controls. Furthermore, among the 14% of errors only 10.8% were due to cytology, whereas 3.6% were due to the punctures. The recent use of prelaparoscopic echography by detecting multilocular cysts should reduce this second percentage.

In 4066 unselected laparoscopies investigated with cytopuncture, 253 cases of intrapelvic endometriosis were disclosed. Of these, 59 (23%) were of pelvic endometriosis with unaffected ovaries, 46 (18%) were of only superficial ovarian endometriosis, 75 (30%) were of endometriotic cysts surrounded by usual stigmata, and 73 (29%) were of unsuspected cysts or intraovarian deposits.

These results show 77% ovarian participation in pelvic endometriosis, one-third of which would have escaped endoscopic diagnosis in the absence of cytopuncture. These results were obtained from a procedure performed during laparoscopy which was almost routine:

(1) The use of a tactile probe needle (Figure 1) which allowed the turning over of each ovary.
(2) The explorative puncture of any fluctuating cortical zone of the ovaries.
(3) The forwarding to an experienced cytologist of every sample no matter how ordinary looking (even serous or yellowish) (Figures 2–4).

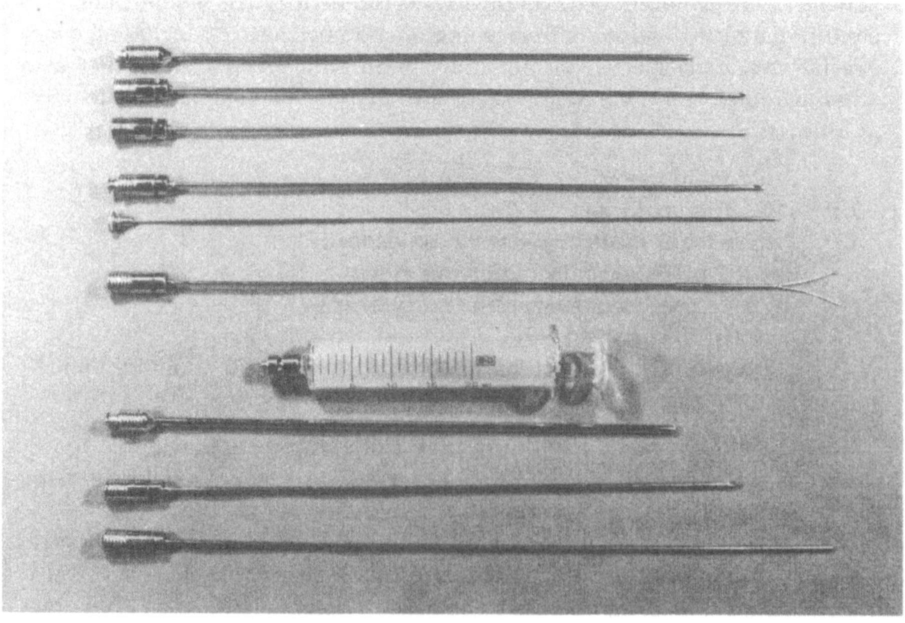

Figure 1 The tactile probe needle. Above the syringe is the 2 mm model, with its mandrels and needle. Below the syringe is the 4 mm model, seldom used, with its mandrels

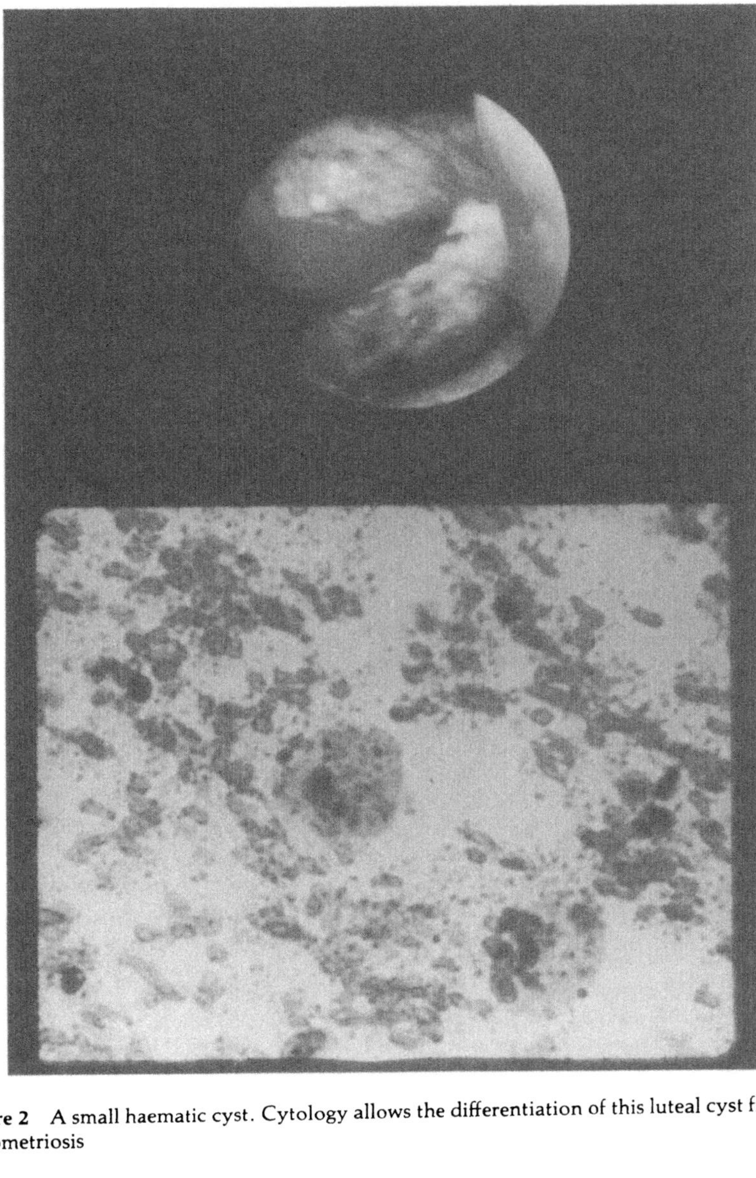

Figure 2 A small haematic cyst. Cytology allows the differentiation of this luteal cyst from an endometriosis

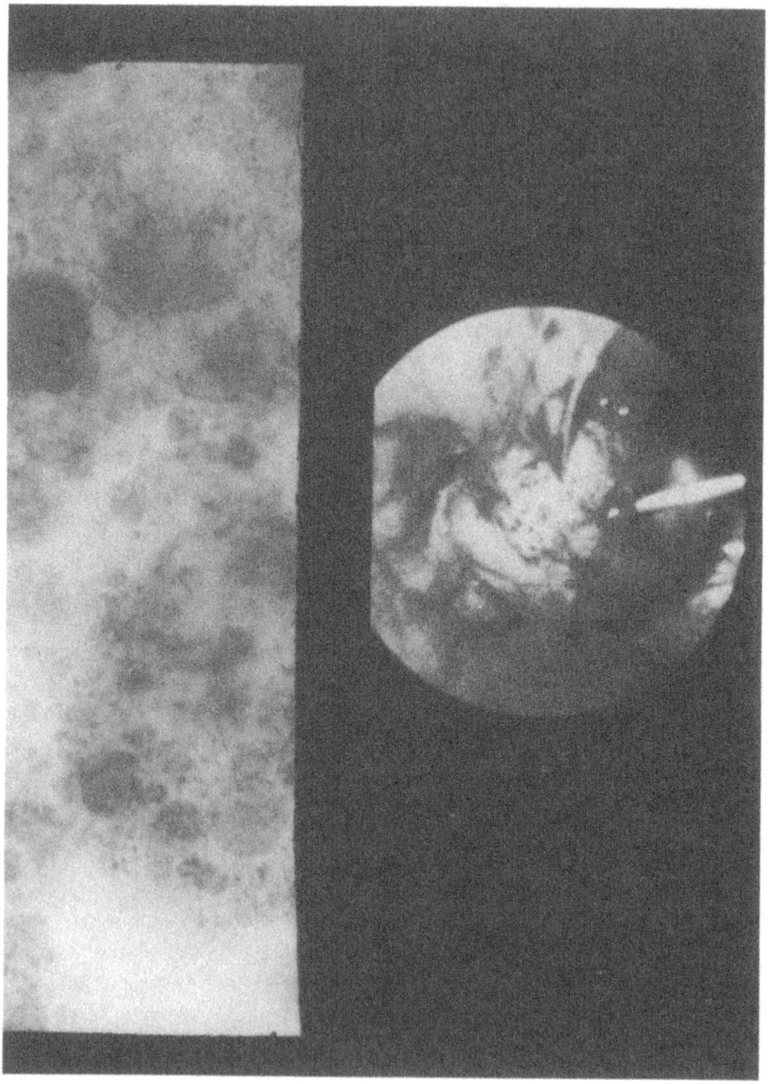

Figure 3 Obvious endometriotic cyst surrounded by haematic adhesions. The sample was chocolate-cream coloured. Cytology shows endometriosis with a large amount of haemosiderin

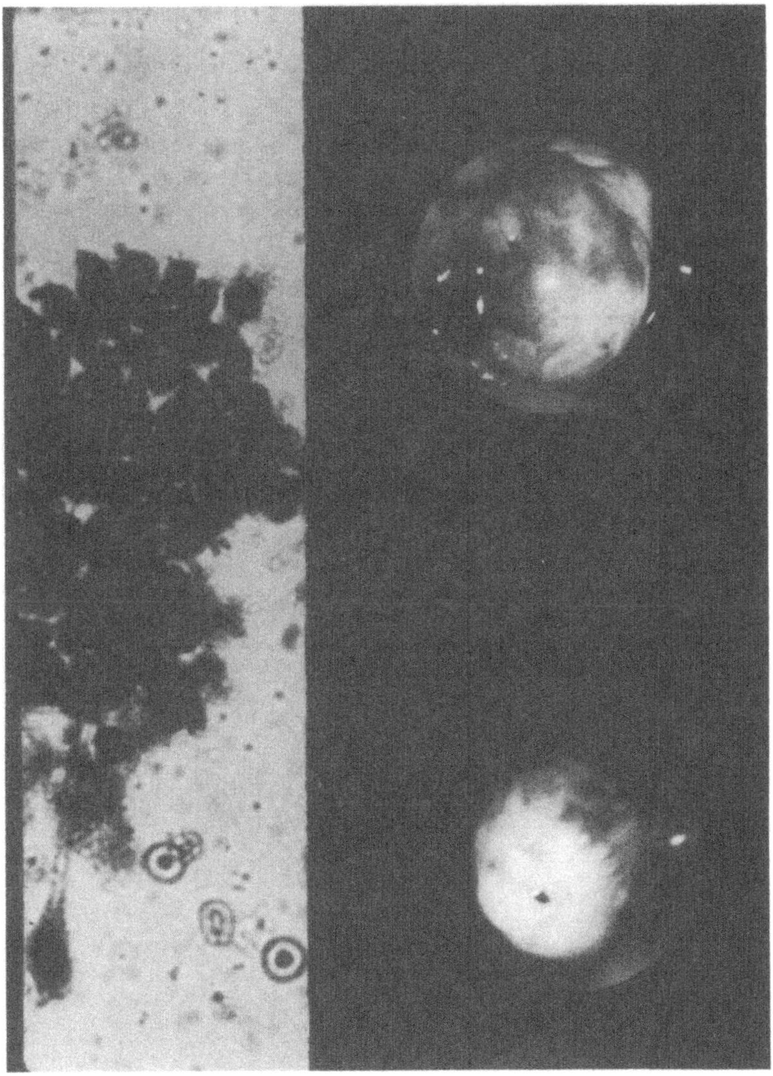

Figure 4 Endometriotic specific signs on non-cystic ovaries. The probe reveals fluctuations. The explorative punture yielded uncharacteristic samples (pink and yellow). Cytology shows fresh endometriosis in both cases

CONCLUSIONS

Explorative intraovarian cytopuncture is essential in endoscopic search of pelvic endometriosis:

(1) To avoid unnecessary endometriotic treatment of haematic luteal cysts.
(2) To detect endometriosis in about 29% of cases of invisible intraovarian deposits.

This should be taken into account in the different international classifications of intrapelvic endometriosis.

Bibliography

Manes, H., Mage, G., Pouly, J. L. and Bruhat, M. A. (1980). Technique, résultats du traitement per-coelioscopique de l'endomètriome ovarien. *Gynecologie*, **31**, 149–52

Mintz, M. and Brux, J. de (1982). Apport de la ponction exploratrice per-coelioscopique et de la cytologie dans le dépistage de 148 cas d'endometriose intraovarienne. *Gynecologie*, **33**, 507–14

Mintz, M., Abeille, J. P. and Audebert, A. (1983). Role de l'aiguille palpateur au cours de la coelioscopie. Utilisation actuelle des explorations instrumentales en gynécologie. Presented at the *XXXI Assises Françaises de Gynécologie*, Caen 12–14 May

Palmer, R., Diquelou, J. Y. and Matuchansly, C. H. (1978). Les résultats comparés de traitements des stérilités avec endomètriose ovarienne. *Gynecologie*, **24**, 33–43

22
Objective assessment of medical treatment of endometriosis with gestrinone (R2323)

J. C. EMPERAIRE and A. J. M. AUDEBERT

Gestrinone (R2323) is a trienic steroid with an ethyl group in position 13, close to norgestrienone which has a methyl group in the same position, and which is marketed in France as a contraceptive pill in association with ethinyl oestradiol (Figure 1). The compound shows an antioestrogenic activity, and a true antiprogesterone activity by competitive binding to the progesterone receptors[1,2].

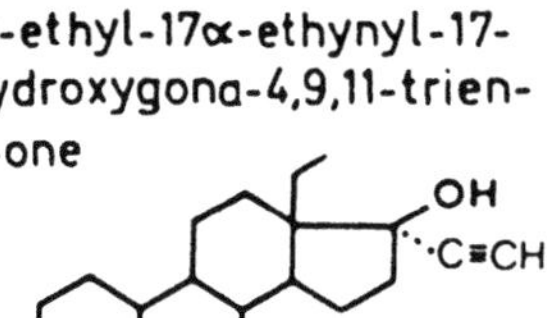

R 2323

13-ethyl-17α-ethynyl-17-hydroxygona-4,9,11-trien-3-one

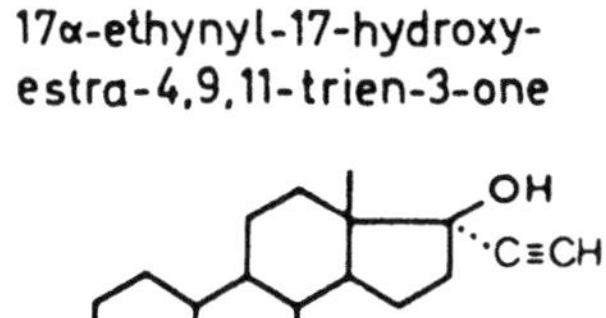

Norgestrienone

17α-ethynyl-17-hydroxy-estra-4,9,11-trien-3-one

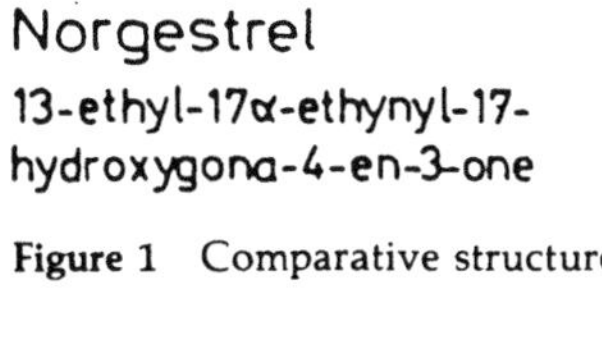

Norgestrel

13-ethyl-17α-ethynyl-17-hydroxygona-4-en-3-one

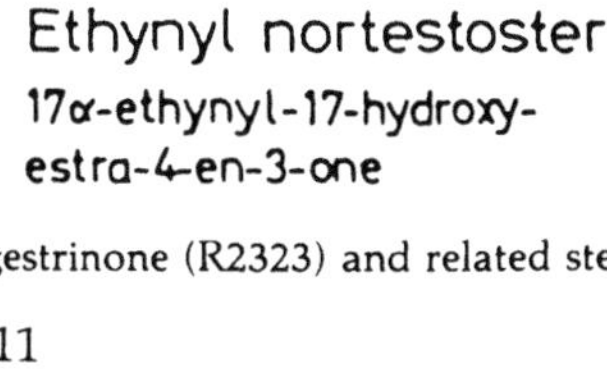

Ethynyl nortestosterone

17α-ethynyl-17-hydroxy-estra-4-en-3-one

Figure 1 Comparative structure of gestrinone (R2323) and related steroids

These antiprogesterone properties result in total antiprogestational, anti-implantation and abortifacient activity in the animal[1]. In the human, gestrinone has so far been extensively studied as a contraceptive agent, but its antiprogesterone activity may be of interest in the medical treatment of conditions such as uterine leiomyomas and pelvic endometriosis[3].

This preliminary study has been devised for objectively assessing the therapeutic effect of gestrinone in pelvic endometriosis associated with painful symptoms and/or infertility.

MATERIALS AND METHODS

Twelve patients have been engaged in the study. All patients, with ages ranging from 24 to 44 years had stage I–III (AFS classification[4]) pelvic endometriosis documented by laparoscopy. They received gestrinone 2.5 mg tablets, one tablet twice a week (total weekly dose 5 mg, six patients) or one tablet three times a week (total weekly dose 7.5 mg, six patients); the therapeutic regimen was not chosen according to the severity of the lesions, but determined at random. All patients were treated for a minimum of 4 months. A monthly evaluation of lipid and carbohydrate metabolism was carried out. A second-look laparoscopy was performed at the end of the treatment.

RESULTS

At the present time, eight among the 12 patients have completed the experimental protocol. The results are shown in Table 1.

The laparoscopic evaluation of pelvic lesions before and after treatment, according to the AFS classification, shows a marked therapeutic effect in all cases but one (number 7); an endometriotic cyst (patient 2) was not affected after 6 months of treatment with gestrinone 5 mg weekly.

The main side-effect was amenorrhoea which developed in all patients but one (number 7); it is interesting that the only patient with poor therapeutic improvement was also the only one to keep bleeding regularly while on therapy. Pertherapeutic spotting affected one patient (number 8), but disappeared when the regimen was temporarily increased to 7.5 mg weekly. The other remarkable side-effect was a weight increase, usually moderate, which in all patients disappeared within 2 months after discontinuation of treatment. Androgenic side-effects were mild. The therapeutic regimen appeared well tolerated, as no patient discontinued the treatment before the expected date.

No variation of glycaemia, total lipids, cholesterol and triglycerides was noted on the monthly evaluations. However, one patient who was borderline hypercholesterolaemic before treatment showed a marked increase in plasma

Table 1 Therapeutic results in eight patients with pelvic endometriosis taking gestrinone, evaluated by pre- and post-therapeutic laparoscopy

No. of patients	*Age* (years)	*Weekly dosage* (×2.5 mg)	*Months of treatment*	*AFS classification of endometriosis*[1] *Before*	*After*	*Weight increase* (kg)	*Other side-effects*
1	24	3	6	29	10	10	–
2	26	2	6	13	8	5	Acne
3	38	2	6	18	4	4	–
4	32	3	4	23	6	0	Mild hirsutism
5	25	3	7	10	5	1.5	–
6	27	3	6	6	1	0	–
7	39	2	8	6	5	2	Regular bleeding
8	44	2	7	3	0	5	Spotting

cholesterol on gestrinone 7.5 mg weekly, which declined to pretreatment values after she was changed to 5 mg weekly.

Follow-up is too short to be significant, but it is noteworthy that one patient (number 3) became pregnant 2 months after discontinuation of treatment.

DISCUSSION

Objective assessment of the therapeutic effect in pelvic endometriosis is possible only by means of laparoscopy. There are many sources of bias in other approaches: appreciation of pain modifications is subjective, and the effect on fertility is also related to other fertility parameters in both partners. Pre- and post-treatment laparoscopic evaluations have already been used for danazol therapy[5].

In this preliminary study, second-look laparoscopy shows that gestrinone is effective on pelvic lesions of endometriosis; however, one case of endometriotic cyst did not show any improvement, but it is well documented that medical treatments are of poor efficiency in the case of endometriotic tumours. This series is too short to determine the respective advantages or shortcomings of both therapeutic regimens, i.e. 5 or 7.5 mg gestrinone weekly.

The main side-effect was pertherapeutic amenorrhoea. In other studies, gestrinone 5 mg weekly was associated with an ovulatory cycle in 44% of patients[6] and a dose of 10 mg weekly did not inhibit ovulation in 15% of the cycles[7]; In most anovulatory cycles, regular menstrual bleeding was noted throughout therapy. This discrepancy with our observations may be due to the fact that in our study gestrinone was given two or three times weekly, whereas in the above-mentioned reports, a single weekly dose was administered. Mild androgenic side-effects were also reported, but the overall clinical tolerance was remarkable with both weekly dosages, as no patient discontinued the treatment.

The biological tolerance was unremarkable. In a study with gestrinone 5 mg weekly, Spellacy *et al.*[8] did not notice any modifications in plasma glucose and insulin on a glucose tolerance test, and no variation of plasma lipids over a 6 month therapeutic period.

CONCLUSION

Many progestogens have previously been used in the medical treatment of endometriosis and danazol has been proposed for the last 10 years as perhaps the most effective agent[5,9]. The efficiency of gestrinone, however, has been objectively documented, and the drug may compare favourably with danazol because of the low dosage required, the few weekly intakes, the good clinical tolerance and the absence of biological side-effects. This preliminary study needs to be completed by a larger series, but gestrinone may represent real progress in the management of endometriosis.

References

1. Azadian-Boulanger, G., Secchi, J. and Sakiz, E. (1971). Biological study of the anti-progesterone effect of R2323. In *Proceedings of the 7th World Congress of Fertility and Sterility*. p. 129. (Amsterdam: Excepta Medica)
2. Sakiz, E. and Azadian-Boulanger, G. (1970). R2323. An original contraceptive compound. In Proceedings of the Third International Congress on Hormonal Steroids. p. 865. (Amsterdam: Excerpta Medica)
3. Coutinho, E.M. (1982). Treatment of endometriosis with gestrinone (R2323), a synthetic anti-estrogen, antiprogesterone. *Am. J. Obstet. Gynecol.*, **144**, 895
4. American Fertility Society (1979). Classification of endometriosis. *Fertil. Steril.*, **32**, 633
5. Dmowski, W.P. and Cohen, M.R. (1978). Antigonadotropin (danazol) in the treatment of endometriosis. *Am. J. Obstet. Gynecol.*, **130**, 41
6. Mora, G., Faundes, A. and Pastore, U. (1974). Clinical evaluation of an oral progestin contraceptive, R2323, 5 mg, administered at weekly intervals. *Contraception*, **10**, 145
7. Victor, A. and Johansson, E.D.B. (1975). The effect of weekly administration of an oral progestogen - R2323 - on the ovarian function. *Contraception*, **12**, 89
8. Spellacy, W.N., Mahan, C.S., Buhi, W.C., Dumbaugh, V.A. and Birk, S.A. (1978). Blood glucose, insulin, cholesterol and triglyceride levels in women treated for six months with the weekly oral contraceptive R2323. *Contraception*, **18**, 121
9. Audebert, A.J.M., Bernard, I. and Emperaire, J.C. (1977). Treatment of endometriosis with danazol. *Gynécologie*, **1**, 29

23
Treatment of infertility due to endometriosis with low-dosage danazol

C. SAMARAS, R. D. GAMBRELL, Jr. and R. B. GREENBLATT

Danazol in dosages of 800 mg daily has been shown to be highly effective in the treatment of endometriosis; however, it may produce significant side-effects[1,2]. Lowering the dosage decreases the number and severity of untoward reactions, and dosages of 100–200 mg daily have been found to be nearly as effective in eliminating endometriosis as dosages of 800 mg[3].

MATERIALS AND METHODS

To determine the lowest effective dosage in treating laparoscopic proven endometriosis, a double-blind study was performed in 27 patients utilizing daily regimens of 0.2, 6.25, 25 and 100 mg danazol for 6 months. During therapy, every patient had monthly exams and the laparoscopy was repeated within 3 weeks of drug completion. The severity of endometriosis was classified into extensive, moderate and minimal. Extensive endometriosis included those with both ovaries enlarged by endometriomas, with involvement of other pelvic organs or bowel. Moderate endometriosis included patients with only one ovary enlarged by endometrioma, small foci present on the contralateral ovary or on other pelvic organs. Minimal endometriosis included small foci on one or more pelvic structures. For comparison purposes, 42 patients with laparoscopic proven endometriosis were treated with menstrual suppression dosages of 400–800 mg danazol daily.

RESULTS

Comparison between the 27 patients in the low-dosage group before danazol 0.2–100 mg daily is made with the 42 patients treated with menstrual suppression dosages in Table 1. There were 15 women classified as suffering

Table 1 Patients treated with danazol for endometriosis

	Low dosage (0.2–100 mg)	*Menstrual suppression* (400–800 mg)
No. in group		
Extent of endometriosis:	27	42
Extensive	6	9
Moderate	8	13
Minimal	13	20
Mean age (years)	29.0±4.37	29.2±3.52
Infertility duration (years)	4.7±2.14	5.8±3.36*
No. (%) symptomatic	8 (29.6)	13 (30.9)
No. (%) with pelvic abnormality	9 (33.3)	11 (26.2)

* Excludes the four women not wishing to conceive.

extensive endometriosis, 21 with moderate, and 33 with minimal disease. With low-dosage danazol, three patients conceived during therapy: two receiving 6.25 mg daily became pregnant after 8 and 15 weeks of medication, and one who conceived while taking 25 mg daily for 5 weeks. The remaining 24 patients had repeat laparoscopy after 6 months of danazol. Progression of endometriosis was evident in three patients at repeat laparoscopy: two treated with 0.2 mg daily and one who had taken 25 mg daily. Improved but persistent endometriosis was found at the second laparoscopy in five women: three treated with 0.2 mg daily, one receiving 6.25 mg daily and one given 100 mg daily. Apparent elimination of endometriosis was the finding in 16 at repeat laparoscopy. To date, 13 of the 27 patients (48.1%) have conceived, including the three who became pregnant during low dosage danazol therapy. Nineteen of the 38 infertile women (50%) treated with 400–800 mg danazol daily have conceived, including one who became pregnant at 7 weeks during therapy with 400 mg daily.

In addition to endometriosis, other associated infertility factors were observed in 43 of the 65 infertile women (66.2%). Oligospermia or a poor postcoital test were the most frequent, occurring in 31 (47.7%), although four patients were anovulatory and four had documented luteal phase defects, including three who also had a poor postcoital test. In patients treated with low-dosage danazol having no other associated infertility factor, 10 out of 13 (76.9%) have conceived while only three of the 14 with other infertility factors

(21.4%) have conceived to date, in spite of every attempt to correct all other factors. Conceptions during or following danazol therapy in the low-dosage group is compared with the conceptions in the menstrual suppression group in Table 2. Where three women received low-dosage danazol conceived during therapy, only one conceived during treatment with 400–800 mg daily. When other infertility factors, in addition to endometriosis, are taken into consideration, 10 of the 13 patients (76.9%) treated with low-dosage danazol have become pregnant, compared with 11 of the 12 patients (91.7%) treated with 400–800 mg daily. In the menstrual suppression group, five out of 10 patients (50%) treated with 400 mg daily have conceived; nine out of 14 women (63.3%) given 600 mg daily have become pregnant; and five out of 14 (35.7%) requiring 800 mg daily have conceived.

Table 2 Pregnancies after different dosages of danazol

	Dosages			
	0.2–100 mg		400–800 mg	
Total conceptions	13/27	(48.1%)	19/38	(50%)
With no other infertility factors	10/13	(76.9%)	11/12	(91.7%)
Extent of endometriosis:				
Extensive	3/3	(100%)	2/2	(100%)
Moderate	4/6	(66.7%)	3/4	(75%)
Minimal	3/4	(75%)	6/6	(100%)

Conception during danazol therapy occurred in five of the 65 infertile women. Since these patients were being followed up at monthly intervals, the pregnancies were diagnosed soon after conception: at 5 weeks' gestation in three and at 4 weeks in the other. The danazol was discontinued as soon as the pregnancy was suspected. All four women were delivered at term with healthy infants, two males and two females. The fifth patient conceived at approximately the time the danazol was increased from 100 to 800 mg daily, when the second laparascopy revealed persistent endometriosis. Unfortunately, the conceptus remained in the fallopian tube and required emergency surgery 4 weeks later to resect the ectopic pregnancy.

Side-effects of danazol therapy were present in both groups; however, 77.8% of the low-dosage group reported no untoward reactions, compared with 54.8% in those treated with 400–800 mg daily. Oedema or weight gain (seven patients) and acne (five patients) were the most frequent complaints, followed by anxiety (four patients) hot flushes (four patients) decreased breast size (three patients) and mild hair loss (two patients). In none of the patients were side-effects severe enough to discontinue the medication. Not only were there much fewer side-effects in the low-dosage group but the complaints were milder than in those treated with 400–800 mg daily and in most cases did not persist through the 6 months of therapy.

DISCUSSION

Danazol, in dosages of 800 mg daily, has been shown to be highly effective in relieving symptoms, resolving implants, and reversing infertility in 55–76% of patients[1]. However, side-effects with 800 mg daily may be significant; so severe in some patients to require discontinuation of danazol[2]. Both the number and severity of untoward reactions are dose related and dosages as low as 100 mg daily may be just as effective[3]. Our data indicate that dosages as low as 6.25 mg danazol daily may be effective in treating endometriosis, regardless of the severity of the disease. Of the 20 patients treated with 6.25 mg or more, the endometriosis was eliminated or conceptions occurred in 18 (90%), while one patient treated with 25 mg had progression of endometriosis, and one treated with 100 mg daily had improvement but persistent endometriosis at repeat laparoscopy.

Only three patients became amenorrhoeic (all on 100 mg daily) on these low dosages of danazol, while 11 out of 27 (40.7%) continued to have regular menses. Therefore, danazol must have an additional action on endometriotic tissue other than menstrual suppression through its antigonadotrophic activity. Confirmation that menstrual suppression is not essential for effectiveness is the fact that three patients conceived during low-dosage therapy, and six others with regular menses during therapy have become pregnant since discontinuation of danazol.

Concern must be expressed for the possibility of fetal abnormalities in patients conceiving during danazol therapy. So far, the four intrauterine pregnancies occurring during danazol treatment progressed normally to term, with births of healthy, apparently normal infants. In Winthrop Laboratories' experience (unpublished observations), 62 pregnant women inadvertently received danazol during pregnancy and 46 were allowed to go to term. All 21 of the males were normal but eight of the 25 females were masculinized (32%). This was limited to clitoral hypertrophy and labial fusion, and all eight mothers had received danazol 800 mg daily until 12–14 weeks' gestation. All of the patients in our low-dosage study were being followed up at monthly intervals, so the danazol was discontinued soon after conception, before major fetal organ systems were developing.

Other infertility factors in addition to endometriosis, or any other factor for that matter, is the sole cause of infertility. Unless these other factors are identified and corrected, conception following successful treatment of endometriosis is unlikely. In conclusion, lower dosages of danazol, 6.25–100 mg daily, may be just as effective as 400–800 mg daily in treating infertility due to endometriosis. Danazol apparently has a direct effect on endometriosis since patients can conceive during low-dosage therapy. Reducing the dosage of danazol reduces the severity of side-effects, and to a lesser extent the number of untoward reactions. In treating patients with infertility, all factors must be evaluated and corrected whenever possible.

Acknowledgements

This study was partially supported by a research grant from Sterling-Winthrop Institute, Rensselaer, New York.

References

1. Greenblatt, R. B., Dmowski, W. P. and Mahesh, V. B. (1971). Clinical studies with an antigonadotropin - danazol. *Fertil. Steril.*, **22**, 102
2. Ansbacher, R. (1975). Treatment of endometriosis with danazol. *Am. J. Obstet. Gynecol.*, *121*, 283
3. Moore, E. E., Harger, J. H., Rick, J. A. *et al.* (1981). Management of pelvic endometriosis with low-dose danazol. *Fertil. Steril.*, **36**, 15

24
Endometriosis associated with hyperprolactinaemia

J. ABE, J. KIMURA, T. TAMAYA
and H. OKADA

INTRODUCTION

We report the serum PRL levels of patients with endometriosis and other various pelvic lesions to clarify as to whether PRL participates in the development and the progression of endometriosis. We also present evidence which suggests that bromocriptine alone or in combination with danazol may be effective for endometriosis.

MATERIALS AND METHODS

The serum PRL levels of 34 patients with endometriosis, 26 patients with adenomyosis, 30 patients with functional dysmenorrhoea and nine patients with myoma uteri were determined by radioimmunoassay measured by Teijin Bio-Science Laboratories (Tokyo, Japan). In this assay system, the normal range for serum PRL level was up to 22 ng ml^{-1} for females. Patients with pituitary adenoma and cases of drug-induced hyperprolactinaemia were excluded from the present study. Thirteen out of 34 cases of endometriosis were classified as Acosta's severe[1] and the remaining cases were graded as Beecham II and III[2]. The serum samples were collected without regard to the menstrual phases. The serum LH and FSH levels of 30 and 99 cases were assayed simultaneously by serum PRL determinations.

The histochemical demonstration of subcellular localization of PRL in normal and ectopic endometria was performed by means of the peroxidase–antiperoxidase method using a PRL Histoset[3] (Immulok Co., Cal., USA).

For assessment of the effectiveness of various drug therapies in endometriosis, we used pelvic computed tomography and hysterosalpingography in addition to bimanual pelvic examinations in some cases.

RESULTS AND DISCUSSIONS

Figure 1 shows the percentage of hyperprolactinaemia in cases with pelvic lesions. The mean (±SD) distribution was 39.0±5.8, 32.8±7.2, 36.4±6.1, 25.9±4.8, 45.8±5.4 in cases of Acosta's severe, Beecham II and III, adenomyosis, functional dysmenorrhoea and myoma uteri, respectively. There were four cases of galactorrhoea in Acosta's severe group, one case in the Beecham II and III groups, two cases in the adenomyosis group and one case in the functional dysmenorrhoea group. Galactorrhoea was not necessarily accompanied by abnormally high serum PRL levels.

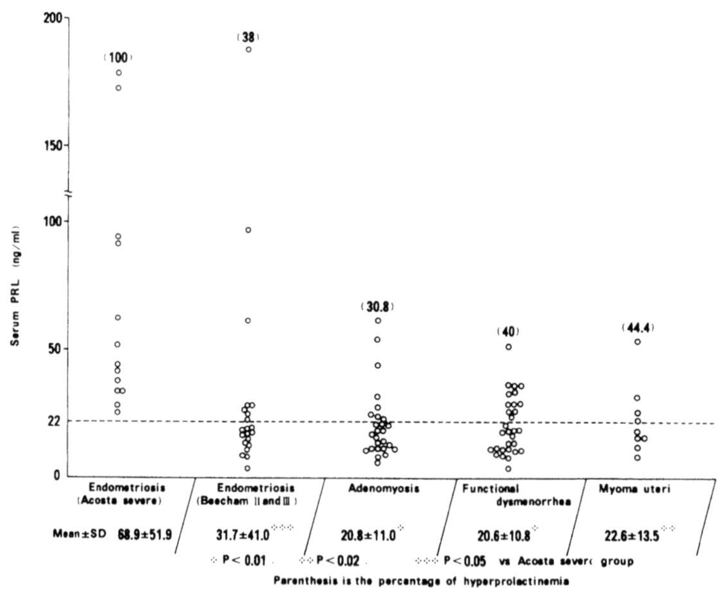

Figure 1 Percentage of hyperolactinaemia in cases with various pelvic lesions

The percentage of hyperprolactinaemia was 100 in Acosta's severe group and that of the other four groups was around 30–40. The mean value of the PRL levels of Acosta's severe cases was significantly higher than that of the other four groups as shown by the *t*-test of significance for unpaired variates.

The mean value of PRL in Acosta's severe group was also significantly higher than that of functional dysmenorrhoea group with hyperprolactinaemia ($p<0.05$). In the Beecham II and III groups, the mean value of PRL was higher than that of adenomyosis, functional dysmenorrhoea and myoma uteri groups but the value was not statistically significant.

As to the correlation between serum PRL and gonadotrophins (LH and FSH), we could not obtain any evidence which indicated that persistently high serum PRL levels markedly increased LH and FSH levels in humans.

The PRL levels in five out of eight cases in the Acosta's severe group fell within the normal range and that of the remaining three cases tended to decrease in 10 days to 6 months after operation, irrespective of the treatment modalities. Normalization of serum PRL level was dependent upon the initial hormone value and the lapse of time after operation rather than the mode of surgery.

The results from the present immunohistochemical study suggests that prolactin acts directly on normal and ectopic endometria, especially on the glandular component (Figure 2).

As it has been already reported elsewhere[4,5], treatments with gestagen or danazol were highly effective for endometriosis. Interestingly, some cases of endometriosis improved symptomatically and objectively by the treatment

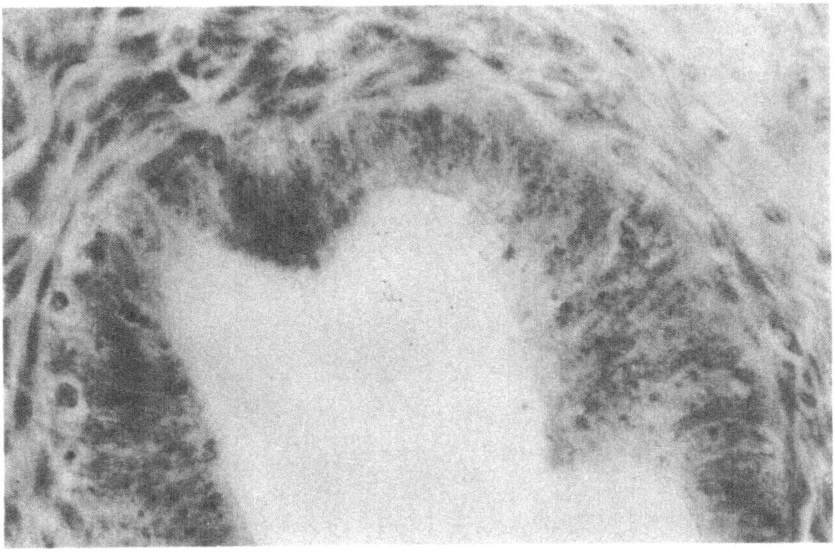

Figure 2 Immunohistochemical demonstration of prolactin binding sites on ectopic endometrium. ×360

with bromocriptine alone. One of four patients judged as a good responder became pregnant after administration of bromocriptine for 2 months. Although it is a small number of cases, the results suggest that bromocriptine alone or in combination with danazol may be effective for endometriosis.

Recently, Mori *et al.*[6,7] successfully induced adenomyosis in mice with intrauterine pituitary isografts and claimed that the development of adenomyosis was primarily dependent upon prolactin and ovarian oestrogen. In the animal model, administration of bromocriptine to mice bearing pituitary isografts completely suppressed the induction of adenomyosis. We demonstrated immunohistochemically the prolactin binding sites on apical glandular membranes in normal and ectopic endometria. This suggests that prolactin may directly act on normal and ectopic endometria in humans, possibly by promoting the development of endometriotic lesions, and that bromocriptine alone or in combination with danazol normalizes abnormal aspects of PRL secretion and consequently suppresses the progression of endometriosis.

References

1. Acosta, A. A., *et al.* (1973). A proposed classification of pelvic endometriosis. *Obstet. Gynecol.*, **42**, 19–25
2. Beecham, C. T. (1966). Classification of endometriosis. *Obstet. Gynecol.*, **28**, 437
3. Sternberger, L. A., *et al.* (1970). The unlabeled antibody enzyme method of immunochemistry. Preparation and properties of soluble antigen-antibody complex (horseradish peroxidase-antihorseradish peroxidase) and its use in identification of spirochaetes. *J. Histochem. Cytochem.*, **18**, 315–33
4. Higashiyama, S. and Okada, H. (1975). Pseudopregnancy in pelvic endometriosis. *Adv. Obstet. Gynecol.*, **27**, 193–202
5. Sakamoto, *et al.* (1982). The clinical effectiveness of danazol for endometriosis. *Sanka to Fujinka*, **11**, 115–38
6. Mori, T., *et al.* (1981). The induction of adenomyosis in mice by intrauterine pituitary isografts. *Life Sci.*, **29**, 1277–82
7. Mori, T. and Nagasawa, H. (1983). Mechanisms of development of prolactin-induced adenomyosis in mice. *Acta Anat.*, **116**, 46–54

25
A newly designed conservative surgery for advanced pelvic endometriosis

O. SUGIMOTO and K. MIYAZAKI

Medical treatment is preferred in the early stage of endometriosis. In advanced endometriosis, however, since the uterus is fixed to the rectosigmoid in retroversion and enlarged, tarry cysts of the ovaries are adherent to the adjacent organs, it is necessary to perform conservative operation as well as hormone therapy.

The hardest procedure of the conservative operation is a peritonization of extensive denudation after lysis of adhesions and a repair of the ovaries after cystectomy.

MATERIALS AND METHODS

During an 11-year period from 1970 to 1980, among 386 infertile patients with pelvic endometriosis, 219 patients underwent conservative operation. For the first 5 years of the series, peritonization and denudation in conservative operation was done by conventional methods such as plication of the adjacent peritoneum or modified Baldy–Webster operation.

In the latter half of the series, we developed a newly devised method in which the peritoneum of both sides of the round ligament was fully used for covering (Figure 1).

The round ligament is transfixed and divided at the insertion of the uterus. The cut end of the round ligament with peritoneal flap is seized and drawn through the loose tissue under the adnexa behind the uterus. The peritoneal flap is stretched and secured over the extensive denuded area.

1

2

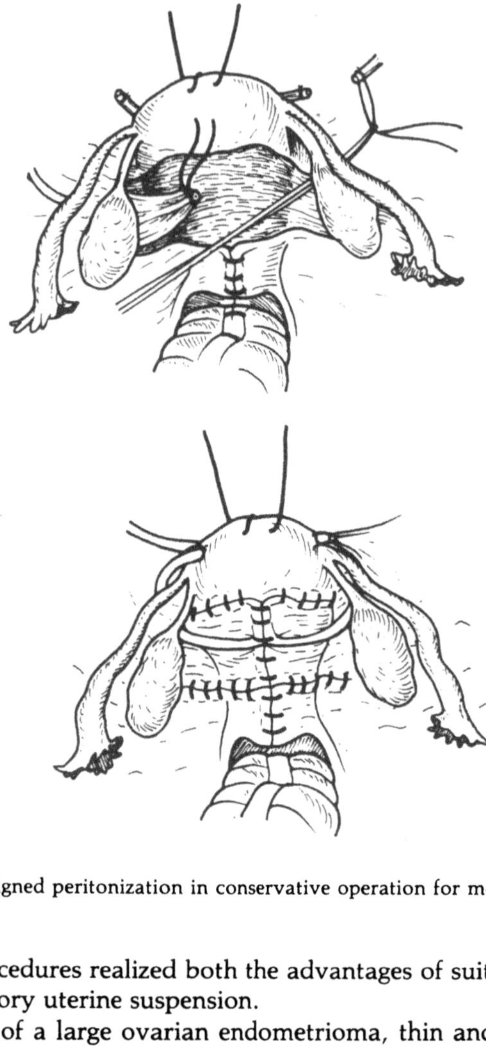

Figure 1 Newly designed peritonization in conservative operation for moderately advanced pelvic endometriosis

Thus these procedures realized both the advantages of suitable peritonization and satisfactory uterine suspension.

After removal of a large ovarian endometrioma, thin and broad ovarian cortex remains. It is a most complicated job to reshape it into the normal ovary contour. The cortex is drawn round and spiral from the hilus to the outside by a purse suture 3–0 Dexon thread on an atraumatic round needle.

The rough edges of the cortex are trimmed. They are cross-stitched by tobacco bag suture.

RESULTS

Conventional operation was attempted in 177 patients, but in 12 of these surgery was inevitably radical because of the limits of its availability (Table 1). The average rate of pregnancy after operation was 47.3%.

Table 1 Conservative and conventional surgical treatment of pelvic endometriosis: outcome

	Extent of disease							
Mode of operation	*Stage I*		*Stage II*		*Stage III*		*Total*	
Conventional*	46		95	(4)	24	(4)	165	(12)
No. (%) of pregnancies	29	(63.0)	41	(43.2)	8	(33.3)	78	(47.3)
Newly designed*	-		6	(50.0)	33	(3)	39	(3)
No. (%) of pregnancies			3	(50.0)	16	(48.5)	19	(48.7)
Total no. of patients*	46		101	(4)	57	(11)	204	(15)
Total no. (%) of pregnancies	29	(63.0)	44	(41.9)	24	(42.1)	97	(47.5)

*No. of patients who underwent radical operation shown in parentheses.

On the other hand, the new operation was attempted in 42 patients with advanced pelvic endometriosis and was successfully performed on 39 patients. The other three patients had to undergo unavoidable radical operation.

Though the new operation performed was limited in the patients with advanced endometriosis, pregnancy rate was almost equal to that of conventional operation which had been done mainly in the cases of stage one and two diseases.

In the group undergoing the new operation, pregnancy occurred within the first year in 14, in the second year in four cases, and another patient conceived in the 4th year after operation. Eventually 19 of the 36 patients became pregnant, but five cases resulted in spontaneous abortion in early pregnancy.

COMMENTS

An attempt was made at a modified Baldy–Webster operation, which was limited to the denuded area. The newly designed operation showed superior results to the conventional methods. It could be successfully performed even in cases of advanced stage and resulted in a high pregnancy rate.

26
Surgical treatment of ovarian endometriosis

M. PEREZ-PELAEZ, A. J. SOBRERO and R. S. JEYENDRAN

Ovarian endometriosis is one of the most fascinating problems encountered in the practice of human reproductive failure. Apparently, Russell of Baltimore[1] was the first to describe ovarian endometriosis. However, the terms endometriosis and endometrioma are attributed to Blair Bell of Liverpool (1922)[2], one year after Sampson[3] described his observations on the 'perforating hemorrhagic (chocolate) cysts of the ovary'.

There have been many attempts at classification of endometriosis which have been met with mixed acceptance. The experience reported here is derived from our private practice, and the cases would be classified as moderate to severe according to Acosta *et al.*[4].

During 3685 laparoscopies performed for the investigation of infertility during the past 7 years we have found 147 cases of ovarian endometriosis of moderate or severe stages; 46 cases were excluded from the present analysis because of other associated pathology that precluded further treatment of infertility, or treatment was refused. Nineteen women were lost to follow-up, discontinuing therapy within 4 months of the surgical intervention; 82 cases remained for analysis.

Symptoms of pelvic endometriosis were present in only 29.7% of the original 147 cases, and in 64.4% the pelvic findings were within normal limits; 15 of the women had been treated previously elsewhere with danazol.

At endoscopy, the most characteristic findings were: collapsed uterus, long utero-ovarian ligaments, hypotrophic or atrophic uterosacrals, ptosed ovaries lying very low in the pelvis, and prominent meso-ovaries. In 67% of the cases the ovaries were bound by adhesions to the broad ligament, and to the uterosacrals in 13.9%.

Where the endometrioma was less than 4 cm in size, endoscopic drainage followed by lavage of the cyst's cavity and the pelvis was performed. When the endometrioma was larger than 4 cm, the women were prepared for laparotomy with norethindrone acetate (5 mg tablets twice daily) for 6–8 weeks in order to create a parenchymal oedema which results in easier and more accurate dissection of the endometrioma.

At surgery, the ovaries were freed from any present adhesions to the neighbouring structures and elevated with stay sutures. On mobilization of the ovaries it is almost always possible to see, near the implantation of the meso, a puckering area surrounding an orifice, often with release of 'chocolate' material. The number and size of the endometriomas vary greatly: in one instance we found 14 endometroid cysts in each ovary; in another, the single structures reached to 14 and 20 cm.

In 84.2% of the cases the ovaries were active and presented luteinized follicles or luteal tissue. The ovarian cortex was very sclerotic in 55.5% of the cases, while in 35.6% it was thick and corrugated.

Surgical treatment consisted of identifying the opening of the endometrioma and with an electric microneedle, a circumoral incision was made in a manner similar to that described more recently by Boeckx *et al.*[5]. In cases where the orifice could not be identified the incision was made in the most protruding part of the cyst or in the antemesomedial portion of the ovary. Once the ovarian cortex was cut, the wall of the endometrioma was shelled out, mostly bluntly and without difficulty, extending the natural cleavage plane, as described by Hughesdon[6], which was always found, and separating the endometriomal wall from the normal ovarian tissue. Any satellite implants were also excised as well as any luteal or luteinized structures. The remaining healthy ovarian tissue was approximated to identify the best direction for reconstructing the organ. Closing was performed with continuous suture of 5-0 polygalactic in two layers: a deep layer for haemostasis and approximation, and one superficial with herring-bone stitches to carefully approach the clean ovarian cortical edges, to prevent adhesions.

The uterosacral ligaments were shortened with non-absorbable suture to elevate the uterus. Similarly, the utero-ovarian ligaments were shortened, anchoring them to the uterine cornua to elevate the gonad, to improve ovarian circulation and to prevent their secondary attachment to previously adherent areas. When the broad ligament was damaged, peritonization was carefully performed stretching the pelvic peritoneum and suturing it with non-absorbable sutures to the posterior aspect of the uterus. We have not encountered the need for grafts.

Following surgery, the patients were treated with a combination of steroids and antibiotics. As soon as menses began, the women received minimal doses of oestrogens and occasionally, when the cervical mucus was optimal, human chorionic gonadotrophin to elicit a better luteal phase.

Sixty-five of the 101 operated women conceived following surgery (64.4%) (Table 1) and of these 12 after laparoscopic surgery alone. Of the 17 women that have not yet conceived six have a major male contributing factor, and of the 15 women treated with danazol 11 conceived after laparotomy with excision of the endometrioma[5].

Table 1 Reproductive outcome of 101 women with ovarian endometrioma treated surgically

	No. of women	*Percentage pregnant*
No. of pregnancies:	65	64.4
Full term	57	87.7
Spontaneous abortion and full term	3	4.6
Spontaneous abortion	4	6.2
Currently pregnant	1	1.5
Non-pregnant	11	10.8
Non-pregnant/severe male factor	6	5.9
Lost to follow-up	19	18.8
Pregnancy rate (%) excluding male factor		79.3
Lost to follow-up		68.4
Lost to follow-up + male factor		85.5

The mean (±SE) time for conception was 7.4±6.5 months; however, over 50% of the conceptions occurred within 6 months of surgery. Where corrugated ovarian cortices were noted, a longer period of post-surgical treatment was required before conception than when sclerotic ovarian capsules were found.

References

1. Russell, W.W. (1899). *Bul. Johns Hopkins Hosp.*, **10**, 8
2. Blair Bell, W. (1922). *J. Obstet. Gynaecol. Br. Emp.*, **29**, 443
3. Sampson, J.A. (1921). *Arch. Surg.*, **3**, 245
4. Acosta, A.A., Buttram, V.C., Jr., Besch, P.K., Malinak, R.L., Franklin, R.R. and Vanderheyden, J.D. (1973). *Obstet. Gynecol.*, **42**, 19
5. Boeckx, W., Gordts, S. and Brosens, I. (1980). Ovarian microsurgery. In Crosigani, P.G. and Rubin, B.L. (eds.) *Microsurgery in Female Infertility*. pp. 59–76. (London: Academic Press)
6. Hughesdon, P.E. (1957). *J. Obstet. Gynaecol. Br. Emp.*, **64**, 481

Part IV

Tubal Factor Diagnosis

Part IV

Section 1
Clinical Results of Diagnostic Endoscopy

27
Laparoscopic findings in 801 sterile patients

C. STADLER, V. MAASSEN, G. POEHNER and M. STAUBER

In the gynaecology department, Berlin-Charlottenburg, we have performed 801 diagnostic laparoscopies in sterile patients between 1962 and 1982. The operation reports were reviewed with special emphasis on tubal pathology and patency. Furthermore, we checked adhesion formation between uterus, tubes and ovaries in order to list all these findings as causes of infertility. We correlated the number of pregnancies with these laparoscopic findings in order to show the prognostic value of laparoscopy in sterility.

The age of the patients varied from 19 to 43 years - the mean value was 29 years. All frequencies were checked with the χ^2 test, with significance at $p<0.05$. Of 801 sterile patients, 531 (66.3%) were diagnosed as suffering from primary sterility and 270 (33.7%) from secondary sterility. The age distribution was as follows: 18–29 years, 381 patients (47.6%); 30–35 years, 347 patients (43.3%); 36–40 years, 66 patients (8.2%); and 40–43 years, seven patients (0.9%).

Adhesion formation - We found adhesions to the uterus in 20% of our patients with a preference for stronger, sail-like adhesions. We registered 14% ovarian adhesions on the right and 13% on the left side. Again, we saw mainly stronger and sail-like adhesions to the ovaries. It seemed interesting that in 5% on the right and in 8% on the left the surface of the ovary was totally covered with adhesions. We were not able to look at the ovaries at all in 4% on the right and in 5% on the left side. Adhesions of the fallopian tubes showed a slight preference, with 32% adhesions on the right and 38% on the left side. On both tubes stronger and again sail-like adhesions were predominant. The fimbrial end showed more alterations by adhesions than the ampulla. The smallest number of adhesions were seen at the isthmus tubae. Table 1 shows the connection between tubal adhesions and other structures of the pelvis. There are *mainly* bindings to the ovary, the pelvis wall and the pouch of Douglas on both sides. There were significantly more adhesions to the intestine – mainly the sigma – on the left side. There was a smaller number of adhesions with uterus, omentum and mesosalpinx.

Table 1 Incidence (%) of adhesions between fallopian tubes and other regions in 801 sterile patients

	Fallopian tube	
Site	*Right*	*Left*
Ovary	56.4	37.8
Pelvis wall	13.4	12.0
Pouch of Douglas	10.6	13.4
Intestine	9.5	23.5
Uterus	5.0	7.4
Omentum	2.8	5.1
Mesosalpinx	2.2	0.9

Pathological findings besides adhesions – We found these in 18% of patients in the ovaries and in 27% in the uterus. The isthmus of the fallopian tube showed pathological findings in 35%, the ampulla in 45%; the fimbrial end was altered in 47% of all cases.

Tubal patency was judged in laparoscopy by the Indigo–Carmine test (Table 2). We found a normal flow of blue dye on the right side in 50.2% and on the left in 51.9% of our cases. A limited flow was seen on the right in 9.2%, on the left in 6.1%. We saw a minimal flow in 2% on the right and 3.2% on the left side. Blue dye was *completely missing* in 23.9% on the right and in 27.8% on the left fallopian tube. A negative test in *both* fallopian tubes was seen in 20.6% of all cases. The patency scale is completed by a number of technical

Table 2 Tubal patency (% of patients) as assessed by Indigo–Carmine test in 801 sterile patients

	Fallopian tube	
Test result	*Right*	*Left*
Normal	50.2	51.9
Limited	9.2	6.1
Minimal	2.0	3.2
Negative	28.6	27.8
Failure	2.6	2.6
Missing	7.4	8.7

failures and a group of patients without an Indigo-Carmine test result in laparoscopy.

Finally, we tried to correlate the number of pregnancies and the primary laparoscopic findings. Laparoscopy was only performed if the examination of the partner showed neither infertility nor severe subfertility. Also, other possible causes of infertility in the *female* patient like cervical dysfunction or anovulation were treated beforehand. Patients with surgical treatment after laparoscopy were excluded from this correlation. Our interest was to show how adhesions *or* other pathological findings in laparoscopy influence the number of pregnancies in previously sterile patients.

In 113 patients we saw a normal situation during laparoscopy and in 38% pregnancies later occurred (Figure 1). If there was an alteration only in one fallopian tube the chances of pregnancy fell to 31%. In 28% pregnancies resulted in a pathological situation in only one ovary. Combined alterations in uterus, tubes and ovaries lowered the pregnancy rate to 14% in this group of patients. Tubal adhesions in both sides lowered the pregnancy rate to 17%; on the other hand, no influence was proved for adhesions on isthmus, ampulla or the fimbrial end.

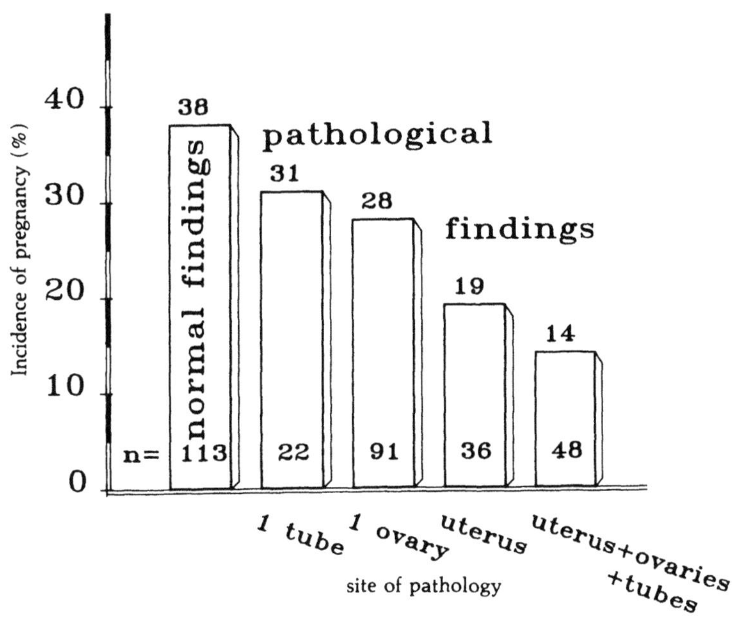

Figure 1 Incidence of pregnancy in patients with normal findings and with pathological findings, according to diagnostic laparoscopy

We have demonstrated a few aspects of our laparoscopic data. After analysis of all findings we intend to summarize them in a new computerized form in order to get clear and more exact information in diagnostic laparoscopy of sterile patients.

28
Improved laparoscopic fertility testing

M. STAUBER, V. MAASSEN, C. STADLER, H. SPIELMANN, M. SCHWERDT, C. DINCER, C. KRUEGER, E. RADKE and R. HARTWIG

Since 1963 more than 3000 couples have been treated in the sterility clinic of the Frauenklinik Charlottenburg at the Free University, Berlin. Treatment and diagnosis covered gynaecological, andrological and psychosomatical aspects of sterility[1]. Up to 1980 laparoscopy was mainly used to evaluate the tubal situation and the anatomy of the pelvis. 27% of the patients showed pathology in the uterus, 35% in the isthmus, 45% in the ampulla, 47% in the fimbria and 18% in the ovaries (see Chapter 25).

After establishing a human reproductive biology laboratory unit[2], the diagnostic spectrum of our laparoscopies could be extended and now also covers ovarian and additional andrological factors. The current concept of improved laparoscopic fertility testing included the following steps:

(1) After hormonal stimulation (e.g. clomiphene 100 mg on days 2–6 of the cycle) the cycle is monitored thoroughly (basal body temperature, cervix score, ultrasound monitoring of follicle size, hormonal analysis).

(2) Application of hCG (e.g. 5000 IU i.m.) according to follicle growth and hormone concentrations: laparoscopy followed 34–36 hours later.

(3) 90–120 min before laparoscopy fractionated homologous insemination (0.1 ml sperm into the cavum uteri and 0.2 ml into the cervix) was performed using a Bourn–Hall catheter.

(4) Throughout laparoscopy the following diagnostic steps are performed:
   (a) Evaluation of the tubal factor (motility, passage, reception of

the ovum) and also of the anatomical situation of the pelvis.

(b) Evaluation of the andrological factor by a modified peritoneal sperm migration (PSM) test[3-5]. This comprises aspiration of peritoneal fluid from the pouch of Douglas (Douglas I), flushing of the adnexa and the pelvis with Ham's f10 and a second aspiration (Douglas II). This is followed by centrifugation of the aspirated fluid according to Ahlgren[6] at 900 *g* for 10 min and examination of the sediment for sperm cells.

(c) Evaluation of the ovarian factor: puncture of mature follicles using the Steptoe needle and also hormonal and cytological examination of the follicular fluid; additionally, histological examination of the follicular wall. If indicated an *in vitro* fertilization test (IVFT) with the husband's sperm is performed. If this is positive, the embryo(s) is replaced.

Figure 1 gives an overview of the whole procedure; this diagram is also used for documentation in our clinic.

The indication for improved laparoscopic fertility testing is given very restrictively. Extensive verbal and written information is provided to both partners. The following criteria are applied for the indication:

(1) Sterility for several years.
(2) Extensive gynaecological and andrological prediagnosis.
(3) No organic or psychological contraindications.
(4) Agreement of both partners to each of the diagnostic steps in a written statement.

PRELIMINARY RESULTS

The number of improved laparoscopic fertility testings ($n=67$) performed by our group is too small so far to show statistically supported correlations. We are therefore reporting some preliminary results which may help to improve individual sterility counselling.

(1) Pathological tubal factors gave indications for microsurgery. Tubal microsurgery was usually timed to allow a simultaneous follicle puncture *in vitro* fertilization.
(2) The peritoneal sperm migration test (PSMT) provided the data shown in Figure 2. A positive PSMT indicates a good chance of conception if there are no additional obstacles. The interpretation of a negative PSM test has to take into account all other diagnostic parameters, e.g. spermiogram, SH test, immunological tests, etc.

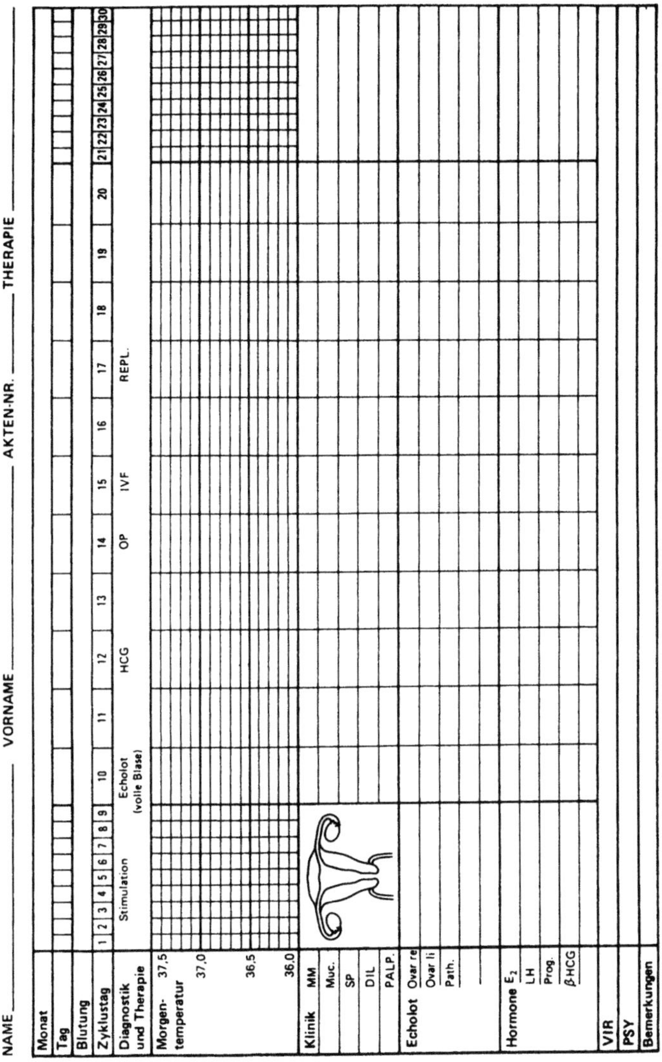

Figure 1 Form used in fertility testing

(3) In most patients one or more oocytes could be obtained using the Steptoe needle. In a few cases atretic follicles, cysts and polycystic ovaries were found and additionally histological examination was used to support the diagnosis 'cyst'. Fertilization resulting in cleavage and replacement could in a few instances be achieved. Patients giving a positive *in vitro* fertilization test can be admitted to an extracorporeal fertilization programme. Staining of granulosa cells from aspired follicles have been used to establish criteria for determining the maturation of oocytes[7].

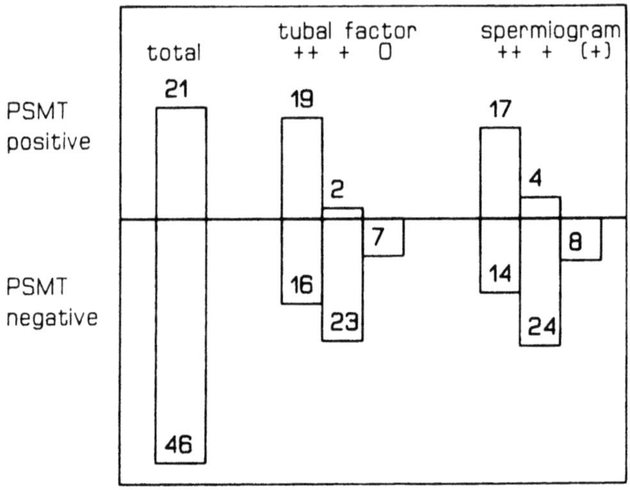

Figure 2 Peritoneal sperm migration test (PSMT) correlated with tubal factor and spermiogram

References

1. Stauber, M. (1979). *Psychosomatik der Sterilen Ehe* (Berlin: Grosse-Verlag)
2. Spielmann, H. (1980). *Die Wirkung von Phenolen in der Praeimplantationsphase der Schwangerschaft am Beispiel von Cyclophosphamid*. PhD Thesis, Free University of Berlin
3. Koch, U. J., Hammerstein, J. and Zielske, F. (1976). Nachweis der Spermatozoenaszension im weiblichen Genitaltrakt als Routineuntersuchung in der Sterilitätsdiagnostik. *Arch. Gynäk.*, **219**, 610
4. Hammerstein, J., Zielske, F., Kratsch, E. and Koch, U. J. (1977). Sperm migration throughout the female genital tract in relation to the time of ovulation. In *The Uterine Cervix in Reproduction*. pp. 238–42. (Bettendorf: Insler)
5. Stamm, J., Campana, A., Maleika, F., Balerna, M., Lucciarini, G. and Archidiacono, A. (1983). Der Peritoneale Spermamigrationstest nach fraktionierter Insemination im Rahmen einer laparoskopischen Fertilitätsabklärung, *Geburtsh. Frauenheilk.*, **43**, 399

6. Ahlgren, M., Boström, K. and Malmquist, R. (1973). *Sperm Transport and Survival in Women with Special Reference to the Fallopian Tube*. pp. 63–73
7. Maassen, V., Stauber, M. and Stadler, C. (1983). Morphologische Untersuchungen an Granulosazellen von punktierten Follikeln im Rahmen des IVFT, XI. Presented at the *Weltkongress für Sterilität und Fertilität*, **26**, June

29
Combined endoscopic findings in 682 infertile women and 135 women requesting sterilization reversal

P. J. TAYLOR, A. LEADER and H. A. PATTINSON

INTRODUCTION

The role of laparoscopy in assessing the reproductive tract of the ovulatory infertile woman is well established. Its superiority to hysterosalpingography (HSG) in the detection of peritoneal and peritubal causes of infertility has been demonstrated in several studies[1-6]. HSG does provide useful information about the uterine cavity not available from laparoscopy. In some instances, the HSG may be either ambiguous or the result difficult to interpret. Hysteroscopy provides a safe method for both the rapid and accurate diagnosis and treatment of many abnormalities of the uterine cavity[2,7,8]. This chapter reports the results of our experience with combined laparoscopy and hysteroscopy in 682 women with otherwise unexplained infertility and 135 women requesting a reversal of sterilization.

PATIENTS AND METHODS

A complete investigation of both partners was undertaken prior to endoscopy[5]. Patients with anovulation or partners with a male causative factor were excluded. Combined laparoscopy and hysteroscopy was performed in 372 women with primary infertility, 282 with secondary infertility and 135 women requesting reversal of a previous sterilization. The procedures were carried out simultaneously under general anaesthesia on a day-care basis as previously described[9]. Dextran 70 (Hyskon, Pharmacia, Piscataway, NJ) was used routinely as the uterine distending medium.

RESULTS

The results are shown in Table 1. Laparoscopy failed in five cases because of patient obesity and subsequent pre-peritoneal emphysema (0.6%). In one case the diagnosis of early pregnancy was made at the time of hysteroscopy and laparoscopy was not undertaken. In one case, a large endometrioma ruptured with insertion of the Verres needle giving a complication rate of 0.3%.

Table 1 Combined endoscopy in 817 women

	Successful	*Failed*	*Complications*	*Total*
Laparoscopy	812	5 (0.6%)	2 (0.3%)	817
Hysteroscopy	793	24 (2.9%)	7 (0.9%)	817
Both procedures	791 (97%)	–	–	817

Aside from the undiagnosed pregnancy (which was considered a failure), the most common cause of hysteroscopic failure resulted from an inability to dilate the cervix. Other causes were: air bubbles in the media and blood obscuring the field of view. There were two cases of uterine perforation and five instances of cervical laceration for a complication rate of 0.9%.

Table 2 Combined endoscopy in 817 women: results

	Laparoscopy normal		*Laparoscopy abnormal*		
Infertility	*Hysteroscopy Normal*	*Hysteroscopy Abnormal*	*Hysteroscopy Normal*	*Hysteroscopy Abnormal*	*Total*
Primary	102	34	152	84	372
Secondary	49	41	102	93	285
Previous tubal	–	–	91	43	134
Grand total					791

Table 3 Most common laparoscopic abnormalities in primary and secondary infertility

	Primary (*n*=372)	*Secondary* (*n*=285)
Periadnexal adhesions	150 (40%)	148 (52%)
Endometriosis	90 (24%)	40 (14%)
Hydrosalpinx	71 (19%)	77 (27%)

The combined endoscopic findings are shown in Table 2. The most common laparoscopic and hysteroscopic findings are shown in Tables 3 and 4.

Table 4 Most common hysteroscopic lesions in primary and secondary infertility, previous sterilization

	Primary	*Secondary*	*Previous sterilization*
Adhesions	60 (16%)*	90 (32%)*†	0 (0%)†
Polyps	48 (13%)	37 (13%)	17 (13%)

* χ^2 test, $p<0.05$.
† χ^2 test, $p<0.05$.

DISCUSSION

Laparoscopy and hysteroscopy have been shown to play an important role in the investigation of the ovulatory infertile woman in several studies[7,10,11]. The combined endoscopic procedures provide complete information on the status of the reproductive tract of these patients while adding little to the operating time.

While laparoscopy in conjunction with HSG is still the most common investigative combination in these cases, consideration should be given to hysteroscopy at the time of laparoscopy. Hysteroscopy is a safe method for the direct, rapid and accurate diagnosis of intrauterine lesions with low failure (2.9%) and complication (0.9%) rates. When others have compared hysteroscopy with HSG, an accuracy rate of 50–62% has been noted for the latter[12]. In this study, intrauterine filmy adhesions were found significantly more often in women with secondary infertility as compared with both primary infertility and women requesting reversal of a previous sterilization. In an earlier paper Taylor and Leader[11] have shown that these adhesions occur independently of intraperitoneal adhesive disease and are related to the occurrence of a previous pregnancy. To what extent these intrauterine filmy adhesions contribute to a patient's infertility is not known. Intrauterine polyps occurred with equal frequency in all women and do not appear to be related to fertility[13].

If hysteroscopic lesions are contributory and perhaps causative of a woman's infertility, then the overall detection rate of 78% for either intrauterine or peritubal lesions or both makes a strong argument for the combined approach. The hysteroscope provides an opportunity not only for detecting intrauterine lesions but also for treating them[2].

References

1. Maathuis, J. B., Horbach, J. G. H. and Van Hall, E. V. (1972). A comparison of the results of hysterosalpingography and laparoscopy in the diagnosis of fallopian tube dysfunction. *Fertil. Steril.*, **23**, 428–31
2. Sugimoto, O. (1978). *Diagnostic and Therapeutic Hysteroscopy*. (Tokyo: Igaku-Shoin)
3. Swolin, K. and Rosencrantz, M. (1972). Laparoscopy *vs.* hysterosalpingography in sterility investigation: a comparative study. *Fertil. Steril.*, **23**, 270
4. Taylor, P. J. (1977). Correlations in infertility: symptomatology, hysterosalpingography, laparoscopy and hysteroscopy. *J. Reprod. Med.*, **8**, 339–42
5. Taylor, P. J. and Cumming, D. C. (1979). Laparoscopy in the infertile female. *Curr. Prob. Obstet. Gynecol.*, **2**, 41
6. Templeton, A. A. and Kerr, M. G. (1977). An assessment of laparoscopy as the primary investigation in the sub-fertile female. *Br. J. Obstet. Gynaecol.*, **84**, 760–2
7. Rosenfeld, D. L. (1978). A study of hysteroscopy as an adjunct to laparoscopy in the evaluation of the infertile woman. In Phillips, J. M. (ed.) *Endoscopy in Gynecology*. pp. 337–40. (Downey, Ca.: American Association of Gynecologic Laparoscopists)
8. Sugimoto, O. (1972). Hysteroscopy. (5) Endometrial polyps. *Obstet. Gynecol. Ther. Jpn.*, **24**, 217–28
9. Taylor, P. J. and Cumming, D. C. (1979). Hysteroscopy in 100 patients. *Fertil. Steril.*, **31**, 301–4
10. Cumming, D. C., Taylor, P. J. (1980). Combined laparoscopy and hysteroscopy in the investigation of the ovulatory infertile female. *Fertil. Steril.*, **33**, 475–78
11. Taylor, P. J. and Leader, A. (1984). Correlations between laparoscopic and hysteroscopic findings in 497 women with unexplained infertility. *J. Reprod. Med.* (In press)
12. Valle, R. (1980). Hysteroscopy in the evaluation of female infertility. *Am. J. Obstet. Gynecol.*, **137**, 425–31
13. Sugimoto, O. (1978). Diagnostic and therapeutic hysteroscopy for traumatic intrauterine adhesions. *Am. J. Obstet. Gynecol.*, **131**, 539–47

Part IV

Section 2
Endoscopic Results in Comparison with other Techniques

30
Diagnostic evaluation of hysterosalpingography in infertile patients

H. IMAIZUMI, R. MORI, S. UEHARA, K. TAKAHASHI,
H. HOSHIAI and M. SUZUKI

From January 1982 to May 1983, we studied 62 cases among the clients of Tohoku University Hospital who were being evaluated for infertility. These clients underwent hysterosalpingography (HSG) and laparoscopy procedures. The purpose of our research was to classify the data obtained by HSG and to correlate that data with findings obtained by laparoscopy.

To perform a HSG for the diagnosis of sterility 38 w/w unctuous contrast fluid is used. Three radiographs were taken: before, at the time, and at 24 hours after contrast fluid injection.

To test for patency of the oviducts by means of laparoscopy, approximately 1.4% methylene blue solution is injected through the cervical os, and the way it flows out through the fimbria is studied.

The data obtained from HSG procedures were classified according to seven structures (Figure 1), while in the laparoscopy they were classified into 13 structures (Figure 2).

In examining the uterine body, of the 62 cases diagnosed as normal by HSG 64.9% were also diagnosed as normal by laparoscopy, and 35.1% as abnormal. Conversely, 68.6% of 35 cases diagnosed as normal by laparoscopy were also judged as normal by HSG and 31.4% as abnormal. These differences might be caused by the different characteristics of the two examination methods; that is, HSG is the method of choice to examine the interior, laparoscopy mainly from the exterior.

In the observations made of the right fallopian tube, of 38 cases diagnosed as

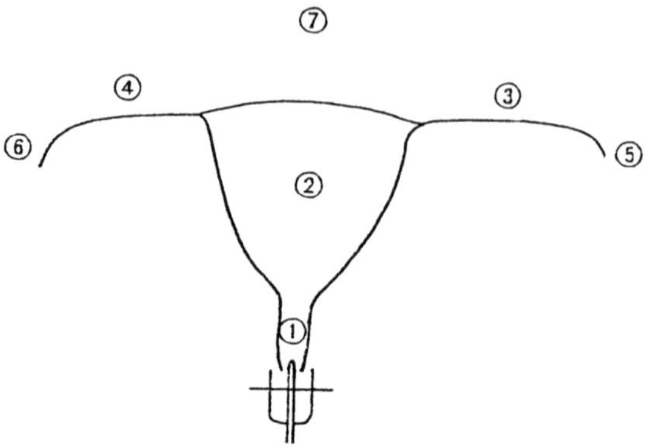

Figure 1 Structures used for classification of HSG findings. 1=Uterine cervix; 2=uterine cavity; 3=left oviduct; 4=right oviduct; 5=left peritoneal tube; 6=right peritoneal tube; 7=peritoneum

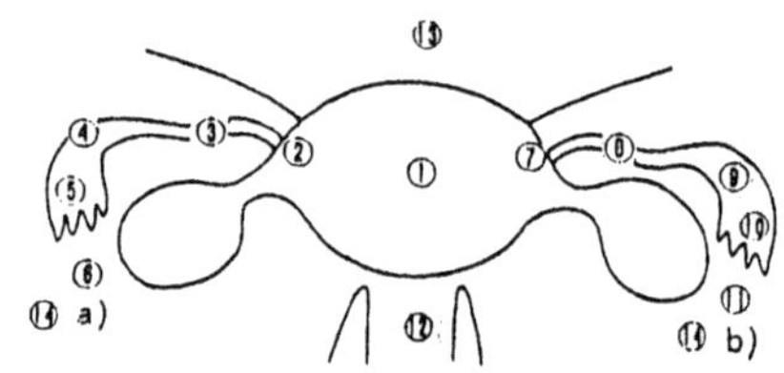

Figure 2 Structures used for classification of laparoscopic findings. 1=Uterine body; 2=left uterotubal junction; 3=left isthmus; 4=left ampulla; 5=left fimbria; 6=left perifimbrillar tube; 7=right uterotubal junction; 8=right isthmus; 9=right ampulla; 10=right fimbria; 11=right perifimbrillar tube; 12=cul-de-sac; 13=peritoneum; 14=patency of the oviduct

normal by HSG 36.8% were judged as normal and 63.2% as abnormal by laparoscopy. Conversely, of 16 cases diagnosed as normal by laparoscopy, 87.5% were normal and 12.5% were abnormal by HSG. In the observation of the left fallopian tube, of 30 cases diagnosed as normal by HSG, 46.7% were judged normal and 53.3% abnormal by laparoscopy. Conversely, of 18 cases diagnosed as normal by laparoscopy, 77.8% were judged normal and 22.2% abnormal by HSG.

These results indicate that HSG is not wholly effective in diagnosing peritubal adhesions, while by laparoscopy it is difficult to locate the occluded part of the oviducts.

We then made comparative studies on the results of the two examination methods concerning the patency of the oviducts. The number of the cases studied was 40. Among them, the number of cases where the evaluation of patency corresponded in both methods was 25, which amounted to 62.5%; the non-corresponding cases amounted to 37.5%. Of these non-corresponding cases, seven were diagnosed as patent by HSG and not patent by laparoscopy. Eight cases were diagnosed as patent by laparoscopy and not patent by HSG.

We classified the results as correlative, non-correlative and unknown and impossible to evaluate.

If, for example, laparoscopic visualization of each structure was not possible, because of partial adhesions, these cases were classified as unknown. If no intra-abdominal observations could be obtained by laparoscopy because of complete intrapelvic adhesions, or if the HSG showed complete closure of both oviducts, these cases were classified as impossible to evaluate (Table 1).

Table 1 Classification of the results between HSG and laparoscopy

Structure	*Correlative*	*Non-correlative*	*Unknown and impossible to evaluate*
Uterine body	31 (50%)	27 (43.5%)	4 (6.5%)
Left oviduct	25 (40.3%)	30 (48.4%)	7 (11.3%)
Right oviduct	25 (40.3%)	31 (50%)	6 (9.7%)
Left peritoneal tube	24 (38.7%)	18 (29.0%)	20 (32.3%)
Right peritoneal tube	25 (40.3%)	18 (29.0%)	19 (30.6%)
Pelvic cavity	21 (33.9%)	27 (43.5%)	14 (22.6%)

From these results we conclude that both HSG and laparoscopy are necessary for the evaluation of infertility. An evaluation based on results of only one of the procedures could lead to a wrong diagnosis.

31
Endoscopy of the tube (tuboscopy): its prognostic value compared with hysterosalpingography

J. HENRY-SUCHET, V. LOFFREDO, L. TESQUIER
and J. P. PEZ

In order to establish a prognosis for tuboplasties, the evaluation of tubal mucosa damage is a major factor, as shown by scanning studies[1]. However, these histological examinations necessitate microbiopsies, usually made at the extremity of the fimbria whose condition may differ from that of the rest of the tube. Hysterosalpingography also gives some idea of the state of the mucosa, particularly if film shots are taken when the tubes are semi-repleted.

A new possibility is to look directly into the tube during the surgery with an endoscope. We propose to call this method tuboscopy. This work compares the information made available by this method to that made available by hysterosalpingography (HSG).

MATERIALS AND METHODS

A tuboscopy was performed during tuboplasties, from January 1980 to September 1982 in 136 cases (231 tubes). Twenty women, with completely normal tubes, undergoing surgery for different reasons, also had a tuboscopy and were used as a control group.

The tuboplasties were made with a Wolf hysteroscope, diameter 4 mm, inclined optique at 60, placed in a casing allowing the adjunction of gas and liquid to the tube, which puts the final diameter at 5 mm.

The supervention of uterine or ectopic pregnancies after surgery was the final control for validation of data.

RESULTS

The different aspects of the mucosa according to tuboscopy are classified into three different groups with sub-groups[2,3]. These different aspects can be observed whatever the exterior of the tube, either normal, stenosed or occluded. They can be associated together.

(1) Normal or subnormal mucosa: the isthmoampullar junction has several folds, regularly distributed which diverge from the isthmus towards the ampulla. In the ampulla, they increase in size, become irregular and in the middle of the ampulla they are covered with numerous, pink, supple villosities which gently move in the tube like seaweed subjected to a current.

(2) Damaged mucosa as a sequela of infectious disease:
   (a) Synechias. These can be of two different sorts: bridge synechias, across the lumen of the tube; or cobweb synechias, papering the tubal wall, sometimes creating one or several internal stenoses (this last aspect is often observed in tubes with chronic chlamydia infection).
   (b) Flat areas. In some parts of the ampulla, the mucosa is flat, smooth, without folds. According to their size and distribution, we can differentiate the following: disseminated flat areas alternating with areas of normal mucosa; flat mucosa with one or two large longitudinal folds; and completely flat mucosa.

(3) Inflammatory aspects. These were observed in three cases. They were considered transitory[3].

COMPARISON BETWEEN HSG AND TUBOSCOPY

This is shown in Table 1. As we compare anatomical findings, we have taken into account the 231 tubes and not the 136 cases. There is a discrepancy between HSG and tuboscopy in an average of 50% of cases. Normal pregnancies (NP) occurred only in women with at least one tube with normal or subnormal mucosa according to tuboscopy, whatever the external lesions and whatever the information given by the HSG. The other women had either ectopic pregnancies (EP) or spontaneous abortions (SA) even in cases where the HSG was normal.

According to the tuboscopy, out of 79 women classified as having normal or subnormal mucosa on best tube, 28 (35%) had uterine pregnancies (UP) and 26

Table 1 Results of tuboscopy compared with those of HSG in 231 tubes*

	(Stenosed tube or adhesions)	*HSG hydrosalpinges*					
Tuboscopy	*Normal mucosa*	*Normal mucosa*	*Irregular mucosa*	*Large folds*	*Flat mucosa*	*Unseen tube*	*Total*
Normal or subnormal mucosa	30 (9np, 1ep, 1sa)	37 (9np, 1sa)	6 (1np)	5 (1np)	4 (1np)	15 (5np, 1ep)	97 (26np, 2ep, 2sa)
Normal mucosa +flat areas	9 (2sa)	12 (2ep)	7	4	3	5	40 (2ep, 2sa)
Abnormal mucosa synechias	11 (2ep)	12 (1sa)	4	1 (1sa)	4 (1ep)	4	36 (3ep, 2sa)
Flat mucosa +1 or 2 folds	0	4 (1ep)	2	7	2	5	20 (1ep)
Flat mucosa	2	4	1	1	22	8	38

np=Normal pregnancy; ep=ectopic pregnancy; sa=spontaneous abortion.
* Results are given as numbers of tubes.

(33%) NP; out of 57 having abnormalities, four (7%) had UP and none had NP; the difference is significant ($p<0.001$). According to the HSG with similar classification, the scores are respectively 23 out of 80 (29%) and 18 out of 80 (22%) if normal folds versus 4 out of 32 (12%) and 3 out of 32 (9%) if abnormal, with no significant difference. The prognostic value of tuboscopy is better.

COMMENTS

These data and similar from Cornier[4] show that tuboscopy has a predictive value of prime importance concerning the prognosis of a tuboplasty. Very simple and easy to perform, it ought to be used as a routine exam during surgery.

The discovery of wide flat areas or multiple synechias seems to indicate such a poor prognosis that if in such cases a longer follow-up does not show normal pregnancies, we will be led to perform bilateral salpingectomies instead of tuboplasties when there are bilateral lesions. In the near future, it seems that *in vitro* fecundation will give these women a better chance of pregnancy.

References

1. Brosens, I., Oberti, C., Vasquez, O., Broeckx, W. and Winston, R. (1977). Ciliated surface of the induct in fertility and infertility. In *Infection et Fecondité*. p. 331. (Paris: Masson)
2. Henry-Suchet, J., Tesquier, L. and Loffredo, V. (1981). Endoscopies tubaires: premiers resultats. *Gynécologie*, **23**, 293
3. Henry-Suchet, J., Tesquier, L., Pez, J. P. and Loffredo, V. (1983). Endoscopie tubaire ou tuboscopie: une exploration complementaire utile dans la chirurgie reparatrice des trompes. In *Utilisation Actuelle des Explorations Instrumentales en Gynécologie*. p. 291. (Paris: Masson)
4. Cornier, E. and Feintuch, M. J. (1984). La fibrotuboscopie ampullaire. (In press)

32
Comparison between uterotubal insufflation, hysterosalpingography and laparoscopy

L. DESSANTI, A. M. S. FOSCOLU, G. B. LA SALA,
C. CIGARINI, G. GHIRARDINI and F. VALLI

The main purpose of this work was to evaluate the reliability of the three more common techniques in tubal patency investigation and to draw conclusions on their single or associated use.

MATERIALS AND METHODS

Our study has taken into consideration 144 patients who came for consultation for sterility lasting longer than 1 year, between October 1981 and December 1982.

In our Division uterotubal insufflation is the first investigation we perform to study the mechanical factors of female sterility. Uterotubal insufflation, hysterosalpingography and laparoscopy with chromopertubation have been performed without the classic contraindications. None of the patients have suffered complications.

For uterotubal insufflation (IUT), the patient was examined in the late follicular phase of the menstrual cycle. The gas used was carbon dioxide at a flow rate of 30 ml min^{-1}. The average duration was 5 min (range 3–9 min).

For hysterosalpingography (HSG), the patient was examined in the late follicular phase. The contrast medium used was a low-viscosity oil (Lipiodol ultrafluid) and the mean quantity used was 6 ml (range 4–10 ml). The radiological technique used was fluoroscopy during the injection of the first 2 ml; thereafter four films were taken.

For laparoscopy with tubal chromopertubation (CCSS) the patient was examined in the early secretory phase and the gas used was CO_2. Double puncture was performed under general anaesthesia. Methylene blue was used for chromopertubation.

There were 144 women. Of these, 70 underwent IUT and HSG, 46 IUT and CCSS, and 28 IUT, HSG and CCSS.

The mean age of the first group (IUT and HSG) was under 35 years. The mean duration of sterility was under 5 years. These patients had not undergone abdominopelvic surgery or suffered from pelvic inflammatory disease (PID); IUDs had not been fitted. Theoretically, these patients have a low risk of mechanical factors of sterility and we decided to perform only the IUT.

The mean age of the group undergoing IUT and CCSS (46 patients) was over 35 years and the duration of sterility over 5 years. Some of the group had undergone abdominopelvic surgery or suffered PID; IUDs had been fitted in some of the women. Theoretically, the risk of mechanical factor is greater in this group than in the first group, and we performed the CCSS immediately after IUT and a HSG later. In both groups the maximum interval between the two examinations was 4 months.

The group undergoing IUT, HSG and CCSS (28 patients) comprised women from couples with idiopathic sterility. Bilateral tubal occlusion was detected by IUT and HSG, there were discordant results for IUT and HSG, difficulty in interpreting IUT and/or HSG, and suspected pelvic adhesions at HSG. The maximum interval between the three examinations was 1 year.

RESULTS

Table 1 shows the results in the group undergoing IUT and HSG. Interestingly, in 11.5% of the cases tubal occlusion by IUT was found to be untrue by HSG.

Table 1 Comparison of the results in the group undergoing IUT and HSG

Results	*No. (%) of patients*
Corresponding IUT and HSG	61 (87)
Tubal patency, IUT-HSG	49 (90.3)
Tubal occlusion, IUT-HSG	12 (19.7)
False-positive IUT	8 (11.5)
False-negative IUT	1 (1.5)

Table 2 presents the results in the group undergoing IUT and CCSS. There is a very high percentage of correspondence between the results of the two examinations and the low percentage of occlusions. However, in the 20% of the patients with tubal patency laparoscopy showed the presence of important pelvic adhesions.

Table 2 Comparison of the results in the group undergoing IUT and CCSS

Results	*No. (%) of patients*
Corresponding IUT and CCSS	44 (95.6)
Tubal patency, IUT–CCSS	41 (93.18)
Tubal occlusion, IUT–CCSS	3 (6.5)
False-positive IUT	1 (2.2)
False-negative IUT	1 (2.2)

Table 3 shows the results in the group undergoing IUT, HSG and CCSS. The number of patients in this group is not high. IUT was discordant, with CCSS in 17.88% of the cases, whereas HSG was discordant with CCSS only in 7.2%. HSG showed two untrue occlusions. In this group the 25% of patients with tubal patency showed important pelvic adhesions.

Table 3 Comparison of the results in the group undergoing IUT, HSG and CCSS

Results	*No. (%) of patients*
Corresponding IUT, HSG and CCSS	22 (78.5)
Tubal patency, IUT–HSG–CCSS	19 (86.36)
Tubal occlusion, IUT–HSG–CCSS	3 (13.64)
IUT discordant *v*. HSG–CCSS	4 (14.28)
False-negative IUT	3 (75)
False-positive IUT	1 (25)
HSG discordant *v*. IUT–CCSS	1 (3.6)
IUT–HSG discordant *v*. CCSS	1 (3.6)

In all patients undergoing IUT and HSG the results of both techniques corresponded in 84 (85.71%) cases and were discordant in 14 (14.29%).

Table 4 comprises the results of IUT and HSG with CCSS. There was no significant difference between the results of IUT and HSG and CCSS. The results of the three examinations corresponded in 90% of the cases.

Table 4 Comparison between the results of IUT, HSG and CCSS in the group undergoing IUT and CCSS and in the group undergoing HSG and CCSS

No. of patients	*Corresponding with CCSS*	*Discordant with CCSS*
IUT 74	67 (90.50%)	7 (9.45%)
HSG 28	26 (92.85%)	2 (7.14%)

CONCLUSIONS

The results of our study show that IUT is a reliable and useful investigation clinically. This is confirmed by the correspondence of the results of IUT, HSG and CCSS in 90% of the cases.

These results justify a delay in using CCSS in the patients with tubal patency at IUT and HSG. They confirm the performance of laparoscopy in cases of discordance between the results of IUT and HSG and indicate the need for laparoscopy in the cases where the history and clinical characteristics of the patients suggest the presence of important pelvic adhesions.

33
Diagnostic laparoscopy in primary infertility

J. PAAVONEN, M. BERG, M. LAHTINEN
and P. K. HEINONEN

INTRODUCTION

Laparoscopy is commonly used in infertility work-up[1]. However, the optimal timing of laparoscopy is not so straightforward. Some prefer performing laparoscopy if other diagnostic tests fail to identify an apparent aetiological factor, whereas some prefer performing laparoscopy early. It is generally known that many infertility factors such as endometriosis and pelvic adhesions are best evaluated by laparoscopy[2]. In this study, we evaluated the laparoscopy results among 113 consecutive women who had primary infertility.

MATERIALS AND METHODS

The study population consisted of 113 consecutive women who had primary infertility and who underwent diagnostic laparoscopy at the Department of Obstetrics and Gynecology, University Central Hospital, Tampere, Finland, 1977–1980. The mean age of the patients was 29.1 years (range 22–39 years) and mean duration of infertility 4.5 years (range 1–14 years). The post-laparoscopy follow-up ranged from 2 to 6 years (mean 3.4 years).

Patient evaluation prior to laparoscopy included determinations of basal body temperature (BBT), serum progesterone, endometrial biopsy, semen analysis and postcoital test (PCT). Hysterosalpingography (HSG) was performed in 102 cases. All test results prior to laparoscopy were normal in 32 patients and those cases were thus considered to be of unexplained infertility.

Laparoscopy plus chromopertubation were performed during general anaesthesia as described elsewhere[1,3]. For pneumoperitoneum 2–5 l of CO_2 was used. Laparoscopy was unsuccessful in five cases.

The sensitivity, specificity and positive predictive values were calculated as described[4].

RESULTS

Table 1 shows the comparison between findings prior to laparoscopy and findings during laparoscopy. Laparoscopy findings were normal in 30 (27%) cases. The most common abnormal laparoscopy findings were endometriosis in 24 (21%) cases, and peritubal adhesions in 35 (31%) cases. Endometriosis was found in 11 (44%) of 25 women in whom it was suspected prior to laparoscopy, and in 13 (15%) of 88 women in whom it was not suspected prior to laparoscopy. Thus the clinical diagnosis of endometriosis had a sensitivity of 46%, specificity of 86% and positive predictive value of 44%.

Table 1 Comparison of findings prior to laparoscopy and during laparoscopy in 113 women who had primary infertility

Finding	*No. (%) prior to laparoscopy*	*No. (%) during laparoscopy*
Endometriosis	25 (22)	24 (21)
Pelvic adhesions	5 (4)	16 (14)
Tubal obstruction	29 (26)	14 (12)
Tubal obstruction and peritubal adhesions	4 (4)	19 (17)
Other factors	18 (15)*	5 (4.5)†
Unexplained infertility	32 (28)	–
Normal	–	30 (27)
Not diagnostic	–	5 (4)

* Hormonal factor, uterine anomaly.
† Polycystic ovaries, fibroid in the uterus.

Among 32 women who had unexplained infertility, endometriosis was found in seven (22%) cases, pelvic or peritubal adhesions in six (19%), tubal occlusion in seven (22%) cases, and only 11 (34%) cases had normal laparoscopy findings.

Table 2 shows the comparison between HSG and laparoscopy in demonstrating tubal occlusion. Of 39 cases with tubal occlusion demonstrated by HSG, only 26 (67%) cases were confirmed by laparoscopic chromopertubation. By contrast, tubal occlusion was demonstrated by chromopertubation in 15 (24%) of 63 cases in whom HSG did not demonstrate tubal occlusion. This last figure is somewhat surprising but it may in part reflect technical difficulties in performing chromopertubation, and in some cases it may be explained by a long time period elapsed since HSG was performed (perhaps subsequent tubal infection had resulted in tubal occlusion). Thus, for HSG in demonstrating tubal obstruction the figures given in Table 2 suggest a sensitivity of 67%, a specificity of 76%, and a positive predictive value of 63%.

Table 2 Comparison between hysterosalpingography and laparoscopy in demonstrating tubal occlusion

Hysterosalpingography (HSG)		*Laparoscopy – occlusion*	
Occlusion	*Number*	*No*	*Yes*
No	63	48	15
Yes	39	13	26
Total	102	61	41

Laparoscopy findings suggesting a post-inflammatory condition (tubal occlusion and peritubal adhesions) were seen in nine of the ten patients who had a history of acute pelvic inflammatory disease (PID), and in 29 (20%) of patients who did not have a history of acute PID, suggesting that pelvic infection frequently is clinically silent.

During the follow-up period, 33 (29%) women became pregnant resulting in 27 live-born babies.

DISCUSSION

We analysed 113 consecutive patients with primary infertility who underwent laparoscopy and found a high rate of abnormal laparoscopy findings such as endometriosis, pelvic and peritubal adhesions and tubal occlusions which were not suspected during the evaluation prior to laparoscopy. The clinical diagnosis of endometriosis was most unreliable. We found endometriosis in 21% overall, and in 22% of those who had unexplained infertility. In fact, only 34% of the patients with unexplained infertility had normal laparoscopy findings. Since endometriosis is one of the most common causes of infertility this suggests that laparoscopy should be performed as a screening test early during the infertility work-up regardless of whether endometriosis was suspected.

Compared with laparoscopy, HSG provides limited information of the presence of peritubal and pelvic adhesions which are one of the most frequent pelvic disorders. We found such adhesions in 31% of the cases. In most cases filmy adhesions between pelvic structures covered large surface areas obviously having impact on fertility.

A spastic tubo-uterine junction may cause false-positive HSG finding. We found that one-third of patients who had tubal occlusion detected by HSG had patent tubes by chromotubation performed during laparoscopy. Thus laparoscopy might even replace HSG as an unnecessary test, though in some cases HSG may provide valuable information on the anatomical abnormalities within the uterine cavity[5] and of regularity of the mucosal outlines of the tubes which is important to know if tubal microsurgery is considered[6]. Therefore infertility laparoscopy and HSG are additive rather than exclusive.

In conclusion, our results suggest that laparoscopy should be used as a screening test as early as possible after the general prerequisites prior to laparoscopy are satisfied.

References

1. Corson, S. L. (1979). Use of laparoscope in the infertile patient. *Fertil. Steril.*, **32**, 359
2. Musich, J. R. and Behrman, S. J. (1982). Infertility laparoscopy in perspective. Review of five hundred cases. *Am. J. Obstet. Gynecol.*, **143**, 293
3. Marik, J. J. (1979). Role of pelvic endoscopy in infertility. *Clin. Obstet. Gynecol.*, **22**, 121
4. Mausner, J. S. and Bahn, A. K. (1974). *Epidemiology: An Introductory Text*. pp. 243–50. (Philadelphia: Columbia Broadcasting System, WB Saunders)
5. Israel, R. and March, C. M. (1976). Diagnostic laparoscopy: A prognostic aid in the surgical management of infertility. *Am. J. Obstet. Gynecol.*, **125**, 969
6. Gomel, V. (1983). An odyssey through the oviduct. *Fertil. Steril.*, **89**, 144

34
Laparoscopy in the investigation of subfertility

P. C. WONG, B. C. OOI, C. ANANDAKUMAR, M. RAUFF
and S. S. RATNAM

INTRODUCTION

For many years, hysterosalpingography has been extensively used in subfertility investigation and is still recognized as one of the most important diagnostic methods. Since Steptoe described the technique of gynaecological laparoscopy in 1967, this endoscopic procedure has been increasingly used as an integral part of the subfertility investigation.

In the University Department of Obstetrics and Gynaecology, laparoscopy was introduced in 1972. Since 1976 it has been used as an integral part in the investigation of subfertility.

MATERIALS AND METHODS

2068 laparoscopies were performed in the years 1976–1981. Of these, 1682 laparoscopies were done as a diagnostic procedure in the investigation of subfertility.

The instrument used was a Wolf 170 degree lens, 10 mm laparoscope. The method was a single-puncture technique described by Steptoe. All cases were performed as in-patients under general anaesthesia. All the patients were sent home on the same day or the day after the operation.

FINDINGS

It was found that the majority of the patients were aged between 21 and 35 years with the peak incidence in the 26–30 age group. This agrees with the national figures that women in Singapore marry at an average age of 24.6 years. Hence if they are still childless at the end of 1 year they will by our definition be classified as subfertile.

Through the laparoscope, a number of aetiological causes of subfertility may be evident, but some factors may not necessarily be the actual cause.

Endometriosis was found in 689 patients or 41.0% of all cases. 387 patients (23.0%) had pelvic adhesions and 192 patients (11.4%) had bilateral blocked tubes due to various reasons. 243 patients (14.4%) had anovulation as evidenced by bilateral smooth ovaries. 17.1% and 24.9% of the patients had polycystic ovaries and retroverted uteri, respectively. Some patients had more than one diagnosis.

Interestingly, only 181 patients or 10.8% of all patients who underwent laparoscopy were found to be normal; that is, the uterus was anteverted, normal, both tubes were patent, both ovaries were normal and scarred, there were no endometriosis or pelvic adhesions.

Endometriosis

The sites of endometriosis found in the 689 cases (41.0%) were as follows: One uterosacral ligament was affected in 163 cases (23.7%) and both uterosacral ligaments in 381 cases (55.3%). One ovary was affected in 63 cases (9.1%) and both ovaries in 47 cases (6.8%); the pouch of Douglas was affected in 243 cases (35.3%). The uterovesical fold was affected in 609 cases (10.0%), there was a unilateral endometriotic cyst in 44 cases (6.4%) and a bilateral endometriotic cyst in 13 cases (1.9%). Some patients suffered endometriosis in more than one site.

The severity of endometriosis was arbitrarily classified as follows:

(1) *Mild* – Only endometriotic spots (regardless of numbers) present, no adhesions and no endometriomas.
(2) *Moderate* – Endometriotic spots (regardless of numbers) present; adhesions present in pouch of Douglas or between ovaries, tubes and uterus; no endometriomas.
(3) *Severe* – Endometriotic spots present, adhesions present, presence of endometrioma(s).

Based on this classification, 540 patients (78.4%) had mild endometriosis whilst 92 (13.4%) and 57 (8.3%) had moderate and severe endometriosis, respectively.

63 patients (9.1%) had bilateral blocked tubes. This is more clearly shown in Table 1 which summarizes the correlation between the severity of endometriosis and tubal blockage.

Table 1 Correlation between severity of endometriosis and tubal blockage in 689 patients*

Severity	*Unilateral* No. (%)	*Bilateral* No. (%)	*Total %*
Mild ($n=540$)	39 (7.2)	42 (7.8)	81 (15.0)
Moderate ($n=92$)	13 (14.1)	16 (17.4)	29 (32.6)
Severe ($n=57$)	3 (5.3)	5 (8.8)	8 (14.0)

* None of the differences were statistically significant.

Pelvic adhesions

Table 2 shows the type of pelvic adhesions found under laparoscopy. 214 cases had adhesions in the pouch of Douglas. Bilateral peritubal adhesions accounted for 43 cases.

Table 2 Pelvic adhesions in 387 patients

Type	*Unilateral*	*Bilateral*
Peritubal	22	43
Between ovary, tube and uterus	40	62
Omentum to ovary, tube and uterus	7	30
Gut to ovary, tube and uterus	10	31
Fimbrial	13	21
Adhesions in pouch of Douglas		214
Adhesions in uterovesical fold		33

Tubal blockage

192 patients (11.4%) had bilateral blocked tubes. Of these, 30 patients had bilateral cornual block and 39 had bilateral fimbrial block. The others were blocked at the isthmus and ampulla. Ninety-five cases had blocks at sites that were not specified.

Tests of tubal patency

Since hysterosalpingography was quite extensively used to test tubal patency, a small study was done to compare the reliability of laparoscopic hydrotubation with that of hysterosalpingography. Forty-two patients who were found to have blocked tubes underwent hysterosalpingography. Of these, 19 cases (45.2%) were in agreement whilst 23 cases (54.8%) were in disagreement.

Table 3 shows the results of another small study. Nineteen subfertile patients whose tubes had been proven to be patent by laparoscopic hydrotubation were included in this study. The hysterosalpingogram was done within the first 5 days following the end of the menstrual period using the FEMCEPT device. A frame-by-frame video-film study of the duration of utero-tubal spasm was recorded.

Table 3 Results of hysterosalpingography in patients with patent tubes on laparoscopy, and on laparoscopy after glucagon

Immediate entry of dye into both tubes	*Entry of dye into both tubes after 60 s*	*Entry of dye into one tube after 60 s*	*No entry of into both tubes after 60 s*	*Failed due to technical difficulties*
		Patent tubes on laparoscopy		
12 (63.2)	1 (5.3)	1 (5.3)	2 (10.5)	3 (15.8)
		Patent tubes on laparoscopy after glucagon		
14 (56)	1 (4)	4 (16)	3 (12)	3 (12)

Out of the 19 patients, only 12 (68.42%) showed immediate entry of dye into and spillage of dye from both tubes. An additional patient showed patency of tubes only after 60 s. One patient showed spillage of dye from one tube after 60 s and in two patients there was no spillage of dye or filling of the tubes even after 60 s. The procedure failed in three patients due to technical reasons. Therefore, patency of tubes was not demonstrated by hysterosalpingography in six out of 19 patients, i.e. 31.57%.

We went further to determine whether the incidence of uterotubal spasm causing apparent tubal occlusion could be reduced with the use of glucagon.

A further 25 patients whose tubes were patent at laparoscopy were recruited. The same procedure of video hysterosalpingography was done but with 2 mg glucagon given intramuscularly 15 minutes before instillation of dye.

Only 14 patients (56%) showed immediate entry of dye into both tubes. Another patient showed fill and spillage from both tubes after 60 s. Four patients showed spillage from one tube after 60 s and another three did not show any even after 60 s. In three other patients the procedure failed for technical reasons. Therefore, 10 patients (40%) had tubal spasm in one or both tubes or failed hysterosalpingography. We concluded that glucagon did not reduce the incidence of tubal spasm during hysterosalpingography.

DISCUSSION

It is interesting to note that in this series, nearly 90 per cent (89.2%) of all the laparoscopies done for investigation of subfertility showed some abnormality. Only 10.8% of all patients were normal. If only hysterosalpingography had been used then only the 195 and 192 patients with one or both tubes blocked respectively would have been identified. 77% of patients with one abnormality or more would not have been identified. This is a strong case to argue for the routine use of laparoscopy in the investigation of subfertility.

Endometriosis was found in 41.0% of all the patients. This appears to be slightly higher than most reported figures[1,2]. Endometriosis seldom causes tubal occlusion. In this series only 9.1% of endometriotic patients had bilateral tubal occlusion and this was not related to the severity of endometriosis. This has been borne out by other authors.

The various tests of tubal patency have been an interesting point of discussion. Most physicians have abandoned the use of tubal insufflation. But there still lies the argument between a hysterosalpingography and laparoscopy. In our series, there was only a 45% agreement between hysterosalpingography and laparoscopy in assessment of tubal patency. Other authors noted agreement figures of 46–78%[3,4]. In our second study, hysterosalpingography failed to show tubal patency in 31.5% of cases. This is to our minds too high a figure and are we would certainly argue for the routine use of laparoscopy in the investigation of a subfertile couple.

References

1. Masson, H.M. (1976). Incidence of endometriosis in diagnostic laparoscopy. *J. Reprod. Med.*, **16**, 135
2. Duignan, N.M., Jordan, J.A. and Coughlan, B.M. (1972). One thousand consecutive cases of diagnostic laparoscopy. *J. Obstet. Gynaecol. Br. Commonw.*, **79**, 1016
3. Swolin, K. and Rosencrantz, M. (1972). Laparoscopy *vs.* hysterosalpingography in sterility investigation. A comparative study. *Fertil. Steril.*, **23**, 270
4. Maathias, J.B., Horbach, J.G.M. and Van Hall, E.V. (1972). A comparison of the results of hysterosalpingography and laparoscopy in the diagnosis of fallopian tube dysfunction. *Fertil. Steril.*, **23**, 428

35
Laparoscopic findings in 375 women attending the Rotunda Hospital Infertility Clinic

P. McKENNA, M. DARLING and R. HARRISON

INTRODUCTION

Tubal pathology is an important and potentially remedial cause of infertility. Laparoscopy is the most accurate method of diagnosis of tubal pathology and can be used to document the extent and aetiology of the problem. In this clinic hysterosalpingography is also used initially if the index of suspicion of tubal pathology is low or if a uterine factor is suspected.

PATIENTS AND METHODS

All patients laparoscoped by one of the three authors in the Rotunda during the study period were eligible to be studied. All infertility patients attending our clinic are laparoscoped unless:

(1) They become pregnant prior to the procedure.
(2) Their husbands have oligospermia.
(3) They have hyperprolactinaemia.
(4) They and their husbands have an unresolved psychosexual problem.
(5) They decline the procedure.

Laparoscopy is done in a standard manner[1] and all procedures are done under general anaesthesia with a cuffed endotracheal tube.

RESULTS

Of the 433 patients laparoscoped the notes of 375 were available for study. Of this total number 262 complained of primary and 113 complained of secondary infertility. The age, range and duration of infertility is shown in Table 1.

Table 1 Mean age of patients and duration of infertility (ranges in parentheses)

Infertility	*Age (years)*	*Duration (years)*
Primary	26 (19–41)	4 (10 months - 13 years)
Secondary	30 (22–38)	3 (6 months - 12 years)

The reproductive profile of these patients is as follows. Sixty-three of the patients had one child, 12 had two children and three had three children. Twenty-four of the patients had suffered a spontaneous abortion, 28 an ectopic pregnancy, and three termination of pregnancy.

Primary infertility – laparoscopic findings

Of the 262 patients with primary infertility 181 were found to have structurally normal pelvic organs. Of the 81 with abnormal findings, 51 were due to previous inflammatory damage, 27 had endometriosis and four had congenital malformations. Of the 51 patients with inflammatory damage the cause was thought to be due to previous pelvic surgery in 24, tuberculosis in two, previous appendix surgery in nine and the cause was unknown, presumed to be pelvic inflammatory disease, in 16.

Secondary infertility – laparoscopic findings

Of the 113 patients with secondary infertility 53 were found to have structurally normal pelvic organs. Of the 60 patients with abnormal findings endometriosis was found in six and inflammatory damage in 54. Of the 54 patients with inflammatory damage previous pelvic surgery (including surgery for ectopic pregnancy) was thought to be responsible in 34 patients whilst the cause was unknown, presumed to be pelvic inflammatory disease, in 20 patients. The results obtained when salpingography is compared with laparoscopy as a method of assessment of tubal patency and pelvic structure is shown in Figure 1.

The results obtained when laparoscopic assessment of ovulation is compared with other methods used to diagnose ovulation (cervical score, plasma progesterone, basal body temperature chart), are shown in Figure 2.

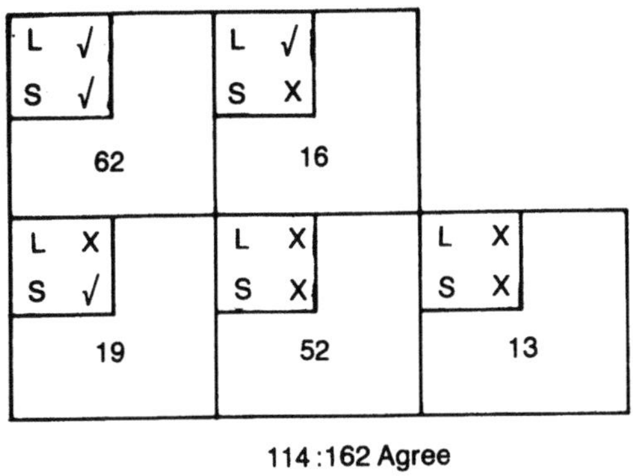

Figure 1 Tubal patency and pelvic structure as determined by laparoscopy (L) and salpingography (S). X=Pathology; ✓=no pathology. U=162

The complications encountered in the 375 laparoscopies were as follows. Nine of the patients suffered minor complications, for which no operative treatment was necessary. These comprised three patients with haemorrhage from the trochar, two with haemorrhage from the pelvis and one with a rectus haematoma. Two patients suffered perforation of uterus and vaginal bleeding was noted in one patient.

Two patients suffered an ovarian haemorrhage after biopsy. These required operative management and were regarded as suffering from a major complication.

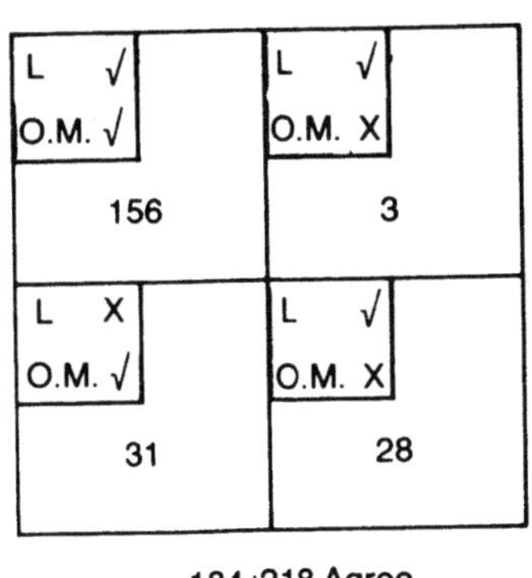

Figure 2 Laparoscopic assessment of ovulation (✓) compared with other methods (OM; cervical score, plasma progesterone and basal body temperature). L=Laparoscopy; X=no ovulation

DISCUSSION

Among the patients attending the clinic one of the more striking features was the long duration of infertility prior to laparoscopy and attendance at the clinic. This is partly explained by the fact that 20% of patients at this clinic are secondary referrals.

When considering laparoscopic findings in the primary infertility group it is of interest that 10% showed evidence of endometriosis. This is in contrast with a figure of 7% that have signs of inflammatory damage that cannot be explained by previous pelvic or appendix surgery or tuberculosis, and pelvic inflammatory disease is the presumed cause. This is in keeping with the low rates of sexually transmitted disease in Ireland.

In the group of patients with secondary infertility, the high rate of previous ectopic pregnancies (25%) is remarkable. This is especially so when considering that the incidence of ectopic pregnancy is much lower in Ireland than in most Western countries[2].

Endometriosis is, as expected, less common in the secondary infertility group (5%) whilst previous pelvic inflammatory disease alone is considerably more common (18%). The comparison of findings made by hysterosalpingography and at laparoscopy has been made previously[3,4]. When we compared the findings in 162 patients (Figure 1) who had both procedures carried out we found agreement in 114 patients. The sources of error are shown and a fifth category (1x:sx) is included. This shows that salpingography indicated pelvic pathology but that this was substantially different from the pathology found at laparoscopy.

In comparing laparoscopic assessment of ovulation with other methods we find a high concordance rate (184:218). This is despite the fact that no attempt is made to time laparoscopy with any particular time of the cycle, other than avoiding menstruation.

Although we would consider laparoscopy as the method of choice in investigating the mechanical factor in infertility we continue to utilize hysterosalpingography mainly because of the small but real risk inherent in laparoscopy and the fact that uterine pathology, including congenital malformations, may best be detected at hysterosalpingography.

References

1. Steptoe, P.C. (1967). *Laparoscopy in Gynaecology*. (Edinburgh: E.S. Livingstone)
2. McKenna, P., Gaughan, B. and Pomeroy, L. (1984). Eleven year survey of ectopic pregnancies in the Rotunda Hospital. *I. J. Med. Sci.* (In press)
3. Coltart, T.M. (1980). Laparoscopy in the diagnosis of tubal patency. *Obstet. Gynaecol.*, **77**, 69
4. Mastroianni, L. (1974). Current concepts in infertility. *Clin. Obstet. Gynaecol.*, **17**, 4

Part V

Microsurgery

Part V

Section 1
Case Selection

36
Contraindications to tubal restorative surgery. Proposal for a dissuasive laparoscopic score

R. PALMER, G. ENAULT and D. SCHMIDT

The contraindications to tubal restorative surgery may be absolute or relative, definitive or temporary. For example, the laparoscopic confirmation of an active persistent inflammatory process is a temporary but imperative contraindication.

Nowadays, it is laparoscopy which allows the final decision. But the decision depends also on the required chances of a pregnancy. We fix them at 20%, and most of the women accept this criterion.

But one must tell them honestly that there is also a risk of extrauterine pregnancy, which in our series is one in four.

For the final decision, some factors which detract (clinical and radiological) also have to be taken into account, for instance age, quality of the husband, habitual anovulation, uterine hypoplasias, synechiae, etc.

LAPAROSCOPIC SCORE

In order to integrate all the laparoscopic factors, we have tried to perfect a laparoscopic score (Table 1).

J. J. Van Assen proposed, in 1976, a simplified scoring system in which each factor (inflammation, adhesions, hydrosalpinx and patency) is graded from 0 to 2 (0=severe lesions; 1=moderate; 2=normal).

For our score, the higher scores correspond to the worst cases.

In fact, we focused our study on a dissuasive laparoscopic score, giving for

Table 1 Means of calculating laparoscopic tubal score

	Right adnexa				*Points*
Patency	1 proximal stenosis	2 distal stenoses	3 proximal occlusion	4 distal occlusion	5 absent
Adhesions	1 moderate	2 extensive	3 dense	4 inflammation	5 frozen
Ampulla	1 small hydrosalpinx	2 large hydrosalpinges	3 thickened wall	4 tuberculosis	5 absent
Isthmus	1 nodular	2 limited destruction	3 extensive destruction	4 absent	
Fimbria	1 hypoplastic	2 partially agglutinated	3 totally agglutinated	4 missing	
Ovary	1 polycystic	2 hypoplastic	3 moderate endometriosis	4 severe endometriosis	5 absent
	Left adnexa – as for right adnexa				
Uterus	1 hypoplastic	2 myomatous	3 malformed	4 synechiae	5 resection
Total	The final score is that of the best side plus uterine score				

each element of the laparoscopic findings a point proportional to the failure rate (that is, the absence of uterine pregnancy), attributable to this element in our personal experience. The failure rate is divided by 20, in order to have all points between 0 and 5.

For instance, in a case of pure proximal occlusion (without adhesions) where a simple cornual anastomosis would give a 60% uterine pregnancy rate, the failure rate would be 40%. The tubal score would be 40/20=2. One should add two points if the fimbria is also partially agglutinated and two if encapsulating adhesions are present on the same side. The total score is that of the best side plus the score for the uterus.

RESULTS

D. Schmidt studied thoroughly 157 consecutive cases laparoscoped by R.P. for an operative decision between June '74 and June '76, with a follow-up of 2–4 years. Among these 137 cases there were:

(1) 104 (66.2%) undergoing immediate operation. These included 27 cases of uterine pregnancy (26%) and six cases of extrauterine pregnancy (5%). In this group, the uterine pregnancies occurred with scores around 7, while in those without uterine pregnancy the scores were around 9. The six cases with extrauterine pregnancy had scores of around 12. No uterine pregnancy was noticed with a score above 11.

(2) Fifty-five (33.8%) who were not operated upon. In 29 cases (18.2%) this was because the lesions appeared too severe. All these cases had scores above 11. No pregnancy occurred in this group. In 24 cases (15.2%) operation was not performed because the lesions did not seem severe enough, and could be cured without operation. Among these were seven cases of uterine pregnancy (29.1%) of which five occurred after per-laparoscopic adhesiolysis, and two were false cornual occlusions. In all of these cases, the score was below 4.

DISCUSSION

Some of our laparoscopies had been performed in cases already known as severe, to convince the patient to give up her quest for an operation. We call these dissuasion laparoscopies.

Nowadays, the situation is different and the laparoscopy of the last chance must also study the chances of an *in vitro* fertilization and embryo transfer and therefore study scrupulously the state of the ovaries and the state of the periovarian adhesions and eventually perform immediately a laparoscopic adhesiolysis of both ovaries, or forecast a surgical adhesiolysis. Every laparoscopy should be followed *immediately* by a very complete report and drawing. We use the chart established by Jeannine Henry-Suchet and distributed by Innothera laboratories, which allows a computerized study.

37
The cytology of tubal secretions for selection of salpingostomies by microsurgical technique

W. ALBRICH, C. PETERS-WELTE, A. GÖTZ and C. HAMMER

Microsurgical procedures have improved the results of reanastamosis considerably[1], whereas the repair of postinflammatory injured tubes has remained disappointing[2]. The intrauterine pregnancy rate after microsurgical salpingostomy lies under 30%, although laparoscopic controls reveal a patency rate of about 90%[3]. This discrepancy leads to the supposition that the degree of damage after PID found in tubal wall and tubal mucosa limits the prognosis of these procedures.

160 of 200 operations performed since 1978 to repair tubal function have a follow-up period of at least 1 year. 57 (35.6%) were salpingostomies. Ten women (17.5%) became pregnant, of which only seven (12.3%) were

Table 1 Morphological classification of hydrosalpinges

Grade	*Tubal wall*	*Proportion of preserved tubal mucosa in the opened infundibulum*
.a	Normal	
.b	Thickened and/or scarred	
I.		75% and more
II.		50%
III.		25% and less
IV.		Intraluminal synechia

intrauterine. The hydrosalpinges were classified according to the preservation of the mucosal surface and fibrotic changes of the tubal wall, as seen through the operating microscope (Table 1).

The prognostic value of this classification can be measured on the experience of 46 salpingostomies (Table 2). Considering this result, one may conclude that operation on hydrosalpinges grades III and IV should be avoided.

Table 2 Classification of hydrosalpinx at salpingostomy, and resulting pregnancies

Hydrosalpinx		*No. of patients pregnant*	
Grade	*No.*	*Intrauterine*	*Ectopic*
I	18	5	0
II	10	1	0
III	15	0	1
IV	3	0	1
Total	46	6	2

In our experience, in contrast to that of other authors[4], hysterosalpingography did not demonstrate the state of the mucosa. On the premise that the cytology corresponded to the degree of damage of the tubal mucosa, the fluid from hydrosalpinges was collected at laparotomy and cytologically examined. After cytocentrifugation, ciliated and secretory epithelial cells, histiocytes,

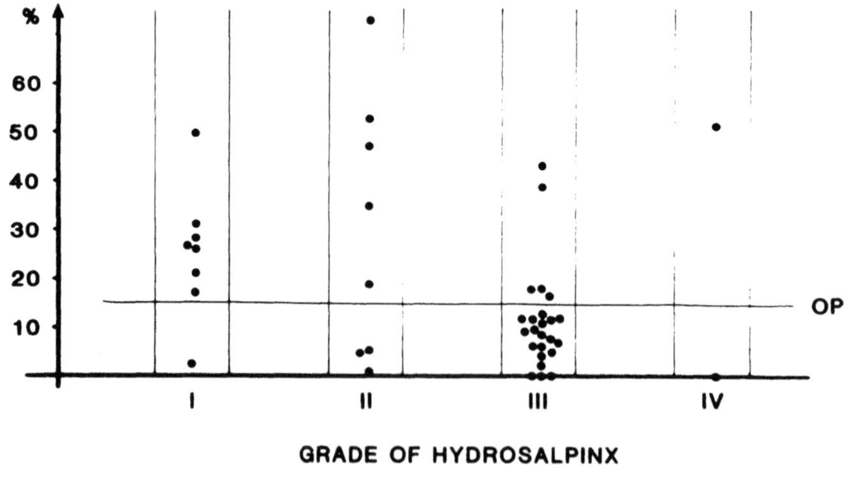

Figure 1 Proportion (as %) of epithelial cells in fluid obtained from hydrosalpinges, according to grade of hydrosalpinx. OP=suggested limit of operability

lymphocytes and leukocytes can be differentiated. Figure 1 shows the proportion of epithelial cells and the morphological classification.

In seven out of the eight cases of grade I hydrosalpinges the epithelial cell rate was over 15%. In five of the eight cases of grade II, this count was also over 15%. There were five false-positive results in the 24 hydrosalpinges of grade III.

To summarize, cytological examination of the fluid from hydrosalpinges showed a rather good correlation with the morphological state found at the opening of the infundibulum. We think, therefore, that cytology may contribute to the decision for or against a salpingostomy.

References

1. Gomel, V. (1980). Microsurgical reversal of female sterilization: A reappraisal. *Fertil. Steril.*, **33**, 587
2. Winston, R. M. L. (1980). Microsurgery of the fallopian tube: From fantasy to reality. *Fertil. Steril.*, **34**, 521
3. DeCherney, A. H. and Kase, N. (1981). A comparison of treatment for bilateral fimbrial occlusion. *Fertil. Steril.*, **35**, 162
4. Young, P. E., Egan, J. E., Barlow, J. J. and Mulligan, W. J. (1970). Reconstructive surgery for infertility at the Boston Hospital for Women. *Am. J. Obstet. Gynecol.*, **108**, 1095

38
In vitro fertilization and embryo replacement in relation to tubal surgery for infertility

P. STEPTOE

The results of *in vitro* fertilization and embryo replacement are now such that the procedure has to be considered when assessments are made of pelvic pathology interfering with ovum pick-up and transport. Assessments of uterine and tubal pathology are best made by hysterosalpingography, hysteroscopy and most importantly by laparoscopy. Laparoscopy will reveal the true extent of extrauterine and extra-tubal pathology, and will allow a good assessment of the operability of tubal and ovarian involvement in former inflammatory or infective lesions. Extrinsic pelvic infections may lead to slight or moderate adhesions without tubal blockage and these are readily removed at laparoscopy. More severe extrinsic infections associated with pelvic or abdominal peritonitis may cause extensive involvement of the internal genitalia in adhesions. The status may require immediate laparotomy to free the ovaries, assess the tubes and decide whether the primary treatment thereafter should be *in vitro* fertilization and embryo replacement.

Intrinsic tubal and tubo-ovarian infections may lead to minimal adhesions with small hydrosalpinges. These might best be treated by surgery to restore tubal patency and function. Anything more severe should now be considered carefully for *in vitro* fertilization and embryo replacement, and any surgical intervention, either by the laparoscope or by the knife should be directed primarily at liberating the ovaries and clearing adhesions for a subsequent oocyte recovery. Large, distorted hydrosalpinges may need removal, but smaller ones often provide a useful structure to manipulate by forceps applied to expose the ovary. Double tubal obstruction - cornual and distal - are now best treated by *in vitro* fertilization and embryo replacement.

ENDOMETRIOSIS

Endometriosis of limited kind is no bar to *in vitro* fertilization and embryo replacement, which indeed is specifically indicated when isthmic pathology is present, or when endometrial cysts of small size are present in the ovary. Preliminary medical treatment may be needed to inactivate the endometriosis, together with laparoscopic destruction of the lesions by thermal coagulation.

PREVIOUS STERILIZATION

Many patients request restoration of their fertility but many have either been sterilized by salpingectomies, removal of ampullae and fimbriae, or by a method that has destroyed much of the tubes. These conditions often render the status inoperable. They are best treated by *in vitro* fertilization and embryo replacement. Where the destruction of the oviducts has been limited then microsurgical techniques may restore tubes of healthy and adequate length and mobility.

PREVIOUS SALPINGECTOMIES

Those associated with ectopic pregnancies are often remarkably clear of pelvic adhesions and are good subjects for *in vitro* fertilization and embryo replacement. Salpingectomies for acute and subacute active infection leave legacies of adhesions which often render access to the ovaries difficult or impossible. Fortunately, one ovary may be reasonably mobile and free, while the other is hopelessly buried. *In vitro* fertilization and embryo replacement is indicated especially with follicular stimulation and ultrasonic identification of the site and number of follicles. When any woman is in the unsatisfied reproductive period of life, her ovaries should be preserved whenever possible, and the surgeon should resist the temptation to remove one of them. Conservative surgery on cysts should be practised whenever possible bearing in mind the possible need for subsequent *in vitro* fertilization and embryo replacement.

Surgical treatment of tubal obstruction is probably to be regarded as a once-only procedure, and if it fails to restore patency the patient should be referred quickly for *in vitro* fertilization. If patency is established, then the infertility should be related to the age of the patient and the passage of time remembering the possibility of *in vitro* fertilization and embryo replacement.

Maybe in the not too distant future we shall see the results of *in vitro* fertilization and embryo replacement bringing about redundancy of tubal surgery altogether.

Such development would certainly be cost effective, since *in vitro* fertilization and embryo replacement can be done much cheaper than tubal surgery once the capital costs and expert teams have been found. It can also be repeated in consecutive cycles, and indeed in many cycles with increasing prospects of ultimate success. Many patients would be relieved of months of psychological stress following tubal surgery.

39
Psychological issues in mechanical infertility

I. EIBSCHITZ, M. ERDREICH, K. DE VRIES, H. SHIHOR
and M. SHARF

Infertility imposes great psychological stress on most couples involved[1]. It was our intention to examine this psychological stress and its influence on the patients in cases of mechanical infertility. The possibility of microsurgical intervention can on the one hand enforce stress and anxiety, but on the other hand hopes can arise by the prospect of the operation that something very drastic can be done to overcome the mechanical barrier to fertility.

PATIENTS AND METHODS

Sixty women with mechanical infertility were evaluated psychologically in a longitudinal study, each of them before and, where possible, after microsurgical intervention. All the women had undergone full infertility work-up, including basal body temperature, progesterone and prolactin evaluation, cervical score, postcoital test, hysterosalpingography and laparoscopy. The husbands had undergone andrological evaluation, including spermograms.

A questionnaire was answered by the women concerning their age, religion, ethnic group, educational level, profession, number of children and years of infertility. Also, the questionnaire included questions about their marital and sexual relations as influenced by the prospect of microsurgical solution of their fertility problems.

The psychological evaluation of the patients was performed by a clinical psychologist. The Crown–Crisp experiential index[2], a modification of the Middlesex Hospital questionnaire, was used to obtain personality profiles on six sub-scale dimensions: free-floating anxiety, phobic anxiety, obsessionality, somatic anxiety, depression and hysteria.

RESULTS

The women interviewed showed, on the whole, evaluated scores on obsessionality, somatic anxiety and depression scales. In a number of cases strong feelings of guilt due to previous abortions, some before the present marriage and without the knowledge of the husband, were found.

The patients received treatment accordingly, i.e. short-term psychotherapy, marital counselling and psychopharmacological support when needed. Nine patients received antidepressive-tetracyclic amine and antianxiety-bromazepam treatment. In one case, a patient from a religious family had an 11-year old son out of wedlock who had been given to adoption, a fact unknown to her present husband. She scored very high on all six sub-scales. Under psychotherapy and antidepressive drug treatment, she decided to tell her husband the truth. Subsequently, her neuroticism score dropped significantly, although her difficult microsurgical operation has not yet led to pregnancy.

Of the 60 women, 45 underwent adhesiolysis as the main microsurgical procedure and 15 salpingostomy. In addition to mechanical problems, artifical insemination by donor was necessary in 12 cases. Nine of the women evaluated become pregnant, one 2 weeks after receiving a child for adoption.

DISCUSSION

There are various causes in the aetiology of infertility. One of them, it seems to us, is psychological stress, even in cases where a mechanical component to infertility seems clearly existent. In many cases, mechanical infertility is secondary to unwanted pregnancies in the past, a fact that by itself may lead to feelings of guilt and tension, which may have their expression in tubal spasm, aggravating the mechanical problem.

Therefore, we advise that all women who are about to undergo microsurgery should be evaluated psychologically prior to the procedure and following it, and the necessary support and treatment should be extended to them, in order to reduce their stress and strain and to enable them to cope and function effectively in their situation, and even with the possibility that the microsurgical intervention may be unsuccessful.

References

1. Menning, B. E. (1980). The emotional needs of infertile couples. *Fertil. Steril.*, **341**, 313
2. Crown, S. and Crisp, A. H. (1966). A short clinical diagnostic self-rating scale for psychoneurotic patients. *Br. J. Psychiatry*, **112**, 917

Part V

Section 2
Special Techniques

40
Danazol as an ovulation inhibitor prior to tubal surgery

L. TESQUIER, J. HENRY-SUCHET, T. LOYSEL, Y. ROBERT
and V. LOFFREDO

INTRODUCTION

The aim of the present study was to demonstrate the usefulness of blocking ovulation before and after tubal plastic surgery. J. Henry-Suchet[1], then Buttram[2], have described the use of such a pre- and postoperative treatment for two reasons:

(1) The surgical act is facilitated: ovariolysis can be done in better conditions, in particular when adhesions are dense and extensive. Ovaries become small and hard with a reduced tendency to bleed.
(2) It prevents postoperative adhesion of the tube to a recent corpus luteum and reduces formation after ovarian surgery of new adhesions. This has been confirmed by a second-look laparoscopy on 8 days post-operatively and has been published earlier[3]. Oestroprogestagens or norethisterone could reach an equivalent result but the thrombo-embolic risk is unacceptable in surgery.

MATERIALS AND METHODS

Since 1980, we have used danazol in 85 cases of tubal plastic surgery with peri-ovarian adhesions in 72 cases. The daily dose has been of 600 mg, given from the first day of menstruation during 4–18 weeks before surgery, and at least 4 weeks after. The mean duration was of 8 weeks.

In a preliminary trial[4] on 20 patients, 600 mg danazol were given for 4–8 weeks prior to tubal surgery. The results show that four patients still had an ovulation. So it was decided to pursue the trial with a longer treatment of at least 8 weeks prior to tubal plastic surgery. In the present trial as in the preliminary one, the ovaries were evaluated during surgery and at early second-look laparoscopy. The drug was considered efficient when no sign of ovarian activity was present. Inefficacy was scored as a semi-failure when there was one follicle but no corpus luteum and as a failure when there were several follicles.

Assays for coagulation parameters were done in 22 patients prior to treatment and after surgery during the danazol treatment. The second assay took place 8 days after the operation. The following were evaluated: thromboplastin platelets, haematocrit, fibrin, factors II, V and VII-X; prothrombin time and activated prothrombin partial time (APPT).

RESULTS

Ovarian inhibition

Table 1 shows that complete inhibition of ovulation was observed in 90% of cases when treatment was given for at least 7 weeks (two semi-failures and one failure out of 30 cases) and 95% if it was for 8 weeks or more (two semi-failures and one failure out of 55 cases).

Table 1 Efficacy of preoperative danazol

Duration of treatment before surgery	*No. of cases*	*Success*	*Semi-failure*	*Failure*
4	3	2	1	0
4–7	27	25	1	1
8–11	47	45	2	0
12	8	7	0	1
Total	85	79	4	2

Recurrence of adhesions

Out of 72 cases with periovarian adhesions before surgery, 8th-day recurrence was observed in 13 patients (18%) and they were bilateral in four cases (5%). The bilateral recurrences were 3.5% if the previous adhesions were velamentous, and 7% if they were dense. This can be compared with a previous series of terminal tuboplasties which included cases with and without ovarian inhibition. These 109 patients had adhesions before surgery, and 27% had a recurrence of new bilateral adhesions on the 8th day.

Side-effects

General tolerance was good. We noticed five cases of weight gain over 5 kg and two cases of acne. There was no arterial hypertension or allergy.

Coagulation findings

The mean of variations before and after danazol (with paired tests) were not significant for most parameters. The variation of platelets, factors VII–X, and an increase in APPT activity were significant, but the figures always stayed within the normal ranges except for one patient who had 800 000 platelets/mm^3 on the second account. However, this last figure was not checked.

COMMENTS

These data show that danazol 600 mg per day given for at least 8 weeks obtains an ovarian inhibition in 95% of cases and that a shorter treatment might be ineffective. Using this method prior to plastic tubal surgery a decreasing rate of recurrent adhesions was obtained versus another series including cases with or without inhibition. As in previous studies[4,5] these results show no significant modifications of most coagulation parameters. The only significant changes we noted on danazol were an increase in factor VII–X levels and APPT activity and also platelets remaining in normal ranges except in one case. These increased rates can be explained by the anabolic effect of danazol or corticoids usually given after the operation; the increases can also be a body reaction after surgery.

This treatment does not seem to expose patients to any thromboembolic risk and might be recommended before and immediately after surgery if there are periovarian adhesions.

References

1. Henry-Suchet, J. and Loffredo, V. (1981). Compared results between two series of terminal tuboplasties. In *GAM Lausanne*. p. 521. Revue médicale de la Suisse Romande.
2. Buttram, V. C., Belue, J. B. and Reiter, R. (1982). Interim report of a study of danazol for the treatment of endometriosis. *Fertil. Steril.*, **37**, 478
3. Henry-Suchet, J. and Loffredo, V. (1982). Techniques d'évaluation des résultats de la microchirurgie tubaire. In Cornier, E. (ed.) *Techniques Microchirurgicales de la Stérilité*. p. 169. (Paris: Masson)
4. Chimbira, T.H., Cope, E., Anderson, B.M. and Bolton, F.G. (1979). The effect of danazol on menorrhagia, coagulation mechanism, haematological indices and body weight. *Br. J. Obstet. Gynaecol.*, **86**, 46
5. Rakoff, A.E. (1976). Side effects of danazol therapy. In Greenblatt, R.B. (eds.) *Recent Advances in Endometriosis*. pp. 108–15. (Princeton, N.J.: Excerpta Medica)

41 Temporary ovarian suspension for prevention of recurrent adhesions after salpingostomy

R. PALMER and E. SEDBON

Recurrent periadnexal adhesions are a major factor of failure after salpingostomy.

Among the numerous methods aimed at their prevention we shall discuss here the temporary suspension of the ovaries, which is a simple, rapid and innocuous complement to the operation.

MATERIAL

The material consists of a series of 165 terminal salpingostomies, operated by R. Palmer between 1960 and 1975. All were done by himself, with the same conventional techniques (Bonney's cuff or Pollosson's racket) and the same peri-operative measures:

(1) When adhesions were absent or discrete, no suspension was performed. This happened in 104 cases (63% of the series).

(2) When an important adhesiolysis was associated with the salpingostomy because of extensive, dense, or vascular adhesions with a zone of deperitonization, a temporary suspension of the ovary was performed, on one or both sides, in 61 cases (37% of the series).

TECHNIQUE

A perfect liberation of the ovary of all adherent remnants must be completed.

The temporary ovaropexy consists in passing a plain 00 catgut through the distal pole of the ovary at 5 mm from its extremity, and then through the peritoneum and subjacent fascia of the pelvic rim, just outside the iliac artery, located by the index finger.

The knot is tied cautiously, to avoid any intrusion of the tube. The whole adnexa is thus lifted at a good distance from the previous zones of adhesiolysis.

Some early control laparoscopies 8 days postoperatively, performed by J. Henry-Suchet, have confirmed that the 00 catgut knot was loosened or loosening by this date.

All our patients had systematically high dosage corticotherapy for 48 hours, beginning the evening before the operation: four ampoules of soludecadron, followed by dexamethasone 3 mg daily for 10–20 days.

RESULTS

(1) In the first group (without ovaropexy), we found among 104 patients,
 37 with at least one intrauterine pregnancy (35.6%),
 27 with at least one living child (21.3%),
 15 with at least one extrauterine pregnancy (14.4%) and 52 without known pregnancy (50%).

(2) In the second group (with temporary ovaropexy), we found among 61 patients,
 15 with at least one intrauterine pregnancy (24.6%),
 13 with at least one living child (21.3%),
 17 with at least one extrauterine pregnancy (27.8%) and
 29 without known pregnancy (47.5%).

A control laparoscopy was performed on 17 patients not yet pregnant 1 or 2 years after the operation, and with persistent patency at hysterosalpingography.

In all of them, the ovary had returned to its normal site. In four cases only some adhesions had recurred.

DISCUSSION

Temporary suspension of the ovaries seems to be a rapid, elegant, innocuous and apparently efficient technique to avoid the recurrence of periovarian adhesions.

The suspended ovary returns habitually to its normal situation probably after 8–15 days at a time when the mesothelial peritoneal layer is reconstituted, avoiding re-coalescence.

But how can we explain the high number of extrauterine pregnancies in this series? These should not be explained by the suspension by itself as laparoscopy demonstrated that ovary and tube had returned to their normal situation in all of the 17 patients controlled.

However, one may think that perhaps a part of the cases with extrauterine pregnancy could be explained by an absence of rapid resorption of the suspension catgut. Unfortunately a large majority of the extrauterine pregnancies were operated far from Paris, and the operator did not mention anything special.

Perhaps the patients in whom we had to perform extensive and laborious adhesiolysis also suffered intratubal synechiae, which were not looked for or treated. The ovarian suspension contributed to the success of the terminal salpingostomy in borderline cases, in which an intratubal pathology was still present.

This is only an hypothesis, but we are convinced that a more critical study of the salpingograms should help to define a group at risk of extrauterine pregnancy after salpingostomy[1].

Another consideration may be in favour of the use of temporary suspension of the ovaries: it is the increasing recourse to *in vitro* fertilization after failure of salpingostomy. The recovery of the ovocytes will be easier, if the ovary is practically free of adhesions.

In order to obtain a constant loosening of the suspension knot, we advise now the use of 0000 (four 0) plain catgut for the suspension, to eventually cut if not loosen it, at control laparoscopy.

CONCLUSIONS

The temporary suspension of the ovary, after a salpingostomy with extensive associated adhesiolysis, seems an effective measure for the prevention of new adhesions.

A doubt remains about its role in the higher incidence of extrauterine pregnancies, as it is not known if the knot had normally loosened in those cases.

In order to obtain a constant loosening of the suspension knot, we now advise the use of 0000 plain catgut for this knot.

References

We have not found in the literature any paper about *temporary* suspension of the ovaries. Some ancient authors quote Poole's ovaropexy, which is done with a linen knot and is definitive.

1. Palmer, R., Proust, ? and Pulsford, ? (1977). Aspect radiographique des trompes chez les femmes stériles ayant fait ultérieurement une G.E.U. *Gynécologie*, **28**, 13

42
Pregnancies after terminal microsurgical tuboplasties with early laparoscopic control on the eighth day

J. HENRY-SUCHET, A. SOLER, F. X. PARIS, J. TORT-GRUMBACH and V. LOFFREDO

Avoiding the recurrence of adhesions after tuboplasty is of prime importance. With this objective in mind, we routinely use microsurgery and early laparoscopy 8 days after operation.

MATERIALS AND METHODS

Out of 241 terminal or bipolar microsurgical tuboplasties, performed in a continuous series from January 1977 to June 1982, 175 primary tuboplasties were reviewed.

Surgical methods

The surgery was carried out using an operative microscope, a microelectrode and nylon 0.6 to 0.8 sutures. Adhesions were carefully removed with a microbistoury; according to previous publications[1] each crude surface was carefully sutured with polyglycolic 0.6 overcasting or treated with free peritoneal grafts when necessary. A temporary tube suspension to the peripheral pelvic wall (catgut 00) is frequently done to prevent the new open tube from glueing itself to the ovary.

Depending on the lesions, five varieties of fimbrioplasties and five of salpingostomies are used.

Fimbrioplasties

(1) Treatment of internal adhesions of the fimbria by using a glass rod with microelectrode.
(2) Treatment of 'classical phymosis'. The stenosed serosa is cut with a microelectrode on its superior edge. The fimbria is turned over on the incision and stitched.
(3) Treatment of 'balloon' phymosis: the terminal part of the ampulla seems to be dilated like a balloon with translucent walls; the fimbria is stenosed. The microscopical observation shows that the 'balloon' is the result of adhesions covering the major part of the fimbria. After incision, the fimbria fringes are carefully removed from the adhesional wall. The fimbria is gently opened, turned over and stitched.
(4) Miscellaneous.
(5) Hydrosalpinges are treated according to Swolin's[2] technique which allows one to obtain a normal or subnormal fimbria with a roughly normal mucosa.

Salpingostomies

In these cases, the opening of the hydrosalpinx showed abnormal (generally flat) mucosa and the tube, after microsurgical opening, was treated, according to classic surgery, in five ways: (1) terminal collar (2) terminal racket, (3) subterminal or medioampullar collar, (4) subterminal or medioampullar racket and (5) miscellaneous.

Early laparoscopy

This was performed 8 days after surgery according to previous publications[3].

Evaluation of results

The patients were classified according to the lesion on the best tube.

(1) Adhesions: if the fimbria is normal. This group includes some cases where the tubes seemed to be occluded according to hysterosalpingography and a previous laparoscopy, but a normal fimbria was revealed after dissection.
(2) Stenoses: usually treated by fimbrioplasties N1 to 4.
(3) Hydrosalpinges: treated either by fimbrioplasty N5 or salpingostomies.

The pregnancy outcome was evaluated in two ways:

(1) Real results are evaluated in 106 cases operated from January 1977 to January 1980 with a 2-year follow-up period, each case without follow-up being considered as a failure.
(2) Cumulative pregnancy rate is evaluated for the whole series (176 cases) according to life tables. Results are considered valid up until a standard variation of $2 \times 10\%$.

For both ways, the first uterine pregnancy of each woman only is taken into account.

RESULTS

'Real' results in 106 cases were as follows. The uterine pregnancy (UP) rate was 49%; 43% if there was hydrosalpinx (60 cases), 48% if stenoses, and 65% if there were only adhesions. The ectopic pregnancy (EP) rate was 9%. Out of the 106 cases, 17 had bilateral laparoscopic adhesiolysis 8 days after surgery. Nine of these women had UP. Therefore, nine out of 52 pregnancies (17%) can be attributed to the early laparoscopy.

The cumulative UP rate was 66% for the whole series, 49% for 96 cases of hydrosalpinges, 43% if there was a stenosis and 44% if there were only adhesions. As these two last groups have the same rate of progress they can be combined, which yields a final result of 55% for both.

COMMENTS

Cumulative pregnancy rate and 'real' results give similar results. The UP rate, (roughly 49% 'real', $66 \pm 2 \times 6\%$ 'cumulative'), is rather high compared with that obtained by other authors.

A possible explanation of this success is the eighth-day adhesiolysis. In previous works[4] we have shown that during a later control, cases with adhesions on the eighth day had the same 20% rate of recurring adhesions as those with no adhesions on the eighth day. The majority of these adhesions were different and due to other causes such as a recurring infection or endometriosis. Trimbos-Kemper and Van Hall[5] had a shorter delay between the operation and the first pregnancy, with fewer ectopic pregnancies, in a series where early laparoscopy was performed compared with the control series. However, a randomized study comprising at least a 2-year follow-up is necessary to demonstrate clearly whether the eighth-day laparoscopy is useful. We have started doing that and the results will be published at a later date.

References

1. Henry-Suchet, J. (1978). Traitement chirurgical des murs adherentiels pelviens. Interêt des greffes peritoneales libres. *Gynécologie*, **2**, 161
2. Swolin, K. (1974). Electromicrosurgery and salpingostomy: long term results. *Am. J. Obstet. Gynecol.*, **121**, 418
3. Henry-Suchet, J. and Loffredo, V. (1978). Prevention de la recidive des adherences au cours des plasties tubaires. I. Interet de la coelioscopie precoce au 8e jour apres la plastie. *J. Gyn. Obstet. Biol. Reprod.*, **8**, 451
4. Henry-Suchet, J. and Loffredo, V. (1981). Techniques d'evaluation des resultats de la microchirurgie tubaire. In Cornier, E. (ed.) *Techniques Microchirurgicales de la Stérilité*. p. 169. (Paris: Msson)
5. Trimbos-Kemper, T. and Van Hall, E. (1984). Second-look laparoscopy after tuboplasty. (In press)

43
Laparoscopic and hysteroscopic CO_2 laser procedures in infertility

Y. TADIR, I. KAPLAN, Z. ZUCKERMAN and J. OVADIA

INTRODUCTION

Laparoscopic and hysteroscopic surgical procedures are routinely used in the treatment of various pathological conditions causing infertility. The revolutionary improvement in optics and lighting, and the development of surgical laser technology, enabled us, a few years ago, to develop our first laparoscopic CO_2 laser prototype[1]. During the past 3 years, modified laparoscopes have been developed by our team and they are routinely used for various indications at several US and European medical centres.

Recently, we developed and tested our first CO_2 laser hysteroscope and preliminary results for lysis of intrauterine adhesions are encouraging.

METHODS

Bearing in mind the potential risks of the laser beam, especially by a 'closed' abdominal approach, special attention was given to assure safety and easy manoeuvrability. Visualization of the abdominal cavity is achieved with the use of the standard 5.8 mm 30 degree Hopkins laparoscope. A second suprapubic 7 mm trocar is used for introduction of the laser cannula.

The instruments presented are modified prototypes which were developed after preliminary experience on animal models and later on humans. These instruments produced by Wolf Endoscopes, West Germany, are made of special stainless steel tubes in various outside diameters with a protecting hook at the distal end, designed to protect adjacent tissues and to grasp the exact tissue selected for dissection (Figure 1). The proximal end is connected to the laser articulated arm with a special 250 mm zinc arcenide focusing lens. The ray is pinpointed by means of coaxial visible helium–neon red light and is centred at the protecting–manipulating hook. For various indications, tubes without this hook are available. An automatic suction, generated synchronously by the main laser instrument foot pedal, collects the smoke produced by tissue vaporization through a special annular channel around the main cannula tubing. This combination allows a clear view in the pelvic area during the procedure, and a clean centre channel for further easy 'lasing'. The interrupted-automatic suction also prevents CO_2 deflation of the abdominal cavity. With this system a third puncture trocar may be used to pass a 5 mm grasping forceps to expose and position pelvic structures. A constant intra-cavity gas pressure is kept using Wisap 'CO_2 pneu automatic', according to Semm.

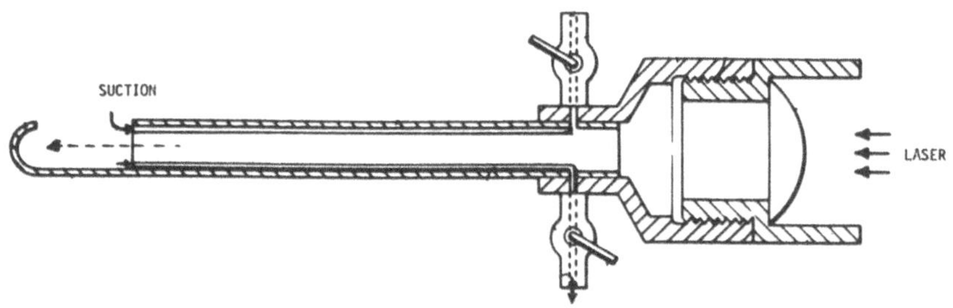

Figure 1 A schematic drawing of the double-puncture CO_2 laser cannula. Protecting hook at the left side. Suction annular channel around the main tubing. Focusing laser lens at the right side

A 12 mm diameter Wolf-operating single-puncture laparoscope with an 8 mm working channel has been modified by an articulated lens and mirror system with a mini-joystick that enables easy focusing of the helium-neon visible light and the laser beam.

Our first laser hysteroscope prototype includes a lens and mirror system, and is designed with three channels: one for the laser beam, one for gas insufflation which improves hysteroscopic visualization, and one for smoke suction.

A vacuum cervical adapter is required in order to make the system leak-proof and a Wolf hysteroscopic insufflator (system Semm) is used to keep intrauterine pressure constant.

A Sharplan apparatus (produced by Laser Industries of Israel) generates the laser beam. Spot size is approximately 0.5 mm and the intensity used is 20–30 W. The laser is fired in interrupted shots of 0.1–0.5 sec or in a continuous mode.

DISCUSSION

Several animal models[2,3] were used to assess the effectiveness of laser microsurgery for adhesiolysis, and other surgeons reported good results performing this procedure in infertile patients with peritubal adhesions[4] and endometriosis[5].

The laparoscopic surgical techniques herein described allow the avoidance of laparotomy in special selected cases such as salpingolysis, avariolysis and mild to moderate endometriosis. Indications have been broadened recently by other surgeons who advocate its use for dysmenorrhoea[6] (destruction of Frankenhauser ganglion), and salpingostomy[7].

Performing the single-puncture technique is a relatively easy and brief procedure provided that the tissues selected for cutting or vaporization are not close to bowel or major blood vessels.

The advantage of the double-puncture technique is that it enables the operator to visualize the abdominal cavity and at the same time to manipulate the laser-operating instrument through a second incision. In addition it offers the possibility of grasping tissue and displacing it independently of the laparoscope. Marking of the helium–neon light is also better.

Table 1 Advantages and disadvantages of laparoscopic CO_2 laser procedures

Advantages	*Disadvantages*
Replace laparotomy in various indications	Expensive and cumbersome instruments
Excision or vaporization of tissue with remote activation	Requires more specific experience
Haemostatic effect during excision or vaporization	Potential risks for adjacent tissues (if not used properly
Thermal-aseptic effect	
Minimal residual tissue destruction effect	
Minimal reformation of adhesions	

The advantages and disadvantages of laparoscopic CO_2 procedures are summarized in Table 1.

Preliminary experience with the hysteroscope for lysis of intrauterine adhesiolysis is encouraging, but as yet it is too early to assess its effectiveness.

In recent years, many pathological condition in various surgical disciplines, mainly plastic, neuro- and general surgery, and various procedures on the uterine cervix have been treated by the CO_2 laser; for this reason laser machines are increasingly available in operating rooms.

The possibility of using the laser laparoscopically may sometimes combine a diagnostic with an operative procedure, especially if the indication for further laparotomy is in doubt.

Contraindications for laparoscopic CO_2 laser procedures are: unsatisfactory viewing of operative field and pathological conditions of bowels or in proximity to ureters, or to blood vessels greater than 1.5 mm.

Although special attention to safety has been undertaken in developing these instruments, it is important to emphasize that their use should be confined to trained laparoscopic surgeons.

References

1. Tadir, Y., Zuckerman, Z. and Ovadia, J. (1981). Laparoscopic CO_2 laser sterilization. Presented at the *Third World Congress of Human Reproduction*, March 22-26, Berlin
2. Tadir, Y., Margara, R., Ovadia, J. and Winston, R.M.L. (1981). Intraperitoneal adhesiolysis by CO_2 laser microsurgery. In *Laser-Tokyo '81*. pp. 13-25. (Inter Group)
3. Scheidel, P., Wallwiener, G. and Pepp, H. (1982). Microsurgical adhesiolysis: a comparative study of the CO_2 and the microelectrode in experimental animals. *Eur. J. Obstet. Gynecol. Reprod. Biol.*, **14**, 55
4. Bellina, J.H. (1981). Microsurgery of the fallopian tube with the carbon dioxide laser, 82 cases with follow-up. In *Laser-Tokyo '81*. pp. 8-3. (Inter Group)
5. Baggish, M. (1981). Intraabdominal application of CO_2 laser for gynecologic surgery. In *Laser-Tokyo '*. pp. 8-1. (Inter Group)
6. Feste, J.R. (1982). Laser laparoscopy – a new modality. In *Proceedings of the Xth World Congress of Gynecology and Obstetrics*. p. 246. (Academy Professional Information Service)
7. Daniell, J.F. (Personal communication)

44
Microsurgical technique for selective removal of tubocornual polyps

S. GORDTS, W. BOECKX and I. A. BROSENS

Philipp and Huber[1] first described the clinical significance of tubocornual polyps but there have been few publications devoted to it since[2-7]. However, the incidence of such polyps on hysterosalpingography is assessed as between 3 and 6%. The diagnosis of tubocornual polyps can be made on routine frontal hysterosalpingography with water-soluble contrast medium. The polyps can be classified as small, medium and large according to Gordts *et al.*[8,9]. The large polyps often have an umbrella-like appearance on the hysterosalpingography. Their base is in the intramural segment but the top of the polyp is protruding in the distended isthmic segment. Spontaneous pregnancies may occur in 30% but large bilateral tubocornual polyps are frequently associated with otherwise unexplained infertility of long duration[7,9]. Grepinet has performed tubouterine implantation in five patients without success because of blockage of the tubes. In the present study a microsurgical technique is described for selective removal of tubocornual polyps.

PATIENTS

Eight patients with long-standing infertility and bilateral large polyps were selected for selective microsurgical polypectomy. The tubes were patent on HSG but showed large defects on both sides at the tubocornual junction. The clinical data related to infertility are shown in Table 1.

Table 1 Clinical data on patients with bilateral large tubal polyps undergoing operation

Duration of primary infertility (years)	*Grade of dysmenorrhoea*	*Associated pathology*	*Intervention*	*Semen analysis*
7	III	Luteal insufficiency	Resection and anastomosis	
5	II	Endometriosis (Acosta I)	Resection and anastomosis, bipolar coagulation, endometriosis	NL
8	0	Endometriosis (Acosta III), fibromatous uterus	Ovarioplasty myomectomy, selective polypectomy	NL
10	II	Endometriosis (Acosta I)	Bipolar coagulation, endometriosis, selective polypectomy	
3	III	Endometriosis (Acosta III)	Ovarioplasty selective polypectomy	NL
3	-	Stein–Cohen–Leventhal syndrome	Bilateral wedge resection, selective polypectomy	NL
6	-	Oligomenorrhoea	Selective polypectomy	NL
6	-	Fibromatous uterus	Myomectomy, selective polypectomy	NL

NL = normal semen: concentration $>20\times10^6$/ml; motility $>50\%$ good motility; morphology $<40\%$ abnormal

MICROSURGICAL TECHNIQUE

Conventional microsurgical instruments and a Zeiss OPMI-6-F operating microscope were used. After routine preparation for microsurgery and transcervical injection of methylene blue the abdomen was opened with a Pfannenstiel incision. With a unipolar micro-electroneedle of 0.2 mm diameter a longitudinal incision of 2 cm is made at the cornu-isthmic junction on the antimesenteric side of the tube.

The endosalpinx was cut longitudinally with a stump curved Castroviejo microdissecting scissor starting the incision on the isthmic part of the tube. After opening the endosalpinx the polyp usually protrudes from the tubal lumen. Further longitudinal splitting of the tube is necessary until the base of the polyp is reached which is mostly deep in the intramural portion. With the stump curved dissection scissors, the polyp is cut at the base. Bleeding is almost absent. Once the polyp is resected, the tube is closed in two layers with separated stitches (nylon 8/0). The first layer includes only the circular muscular layer and the second layer the serosa and subserosal longitudinal muscular layer.

RESULTS

Before attempting selective microsurgical polypectomy two patients were operated with resection of the tubocornual segment and the implantation basis of the polyp followed by deep tubocornual anastomosis.

However, subsequent hysterosalpingography showed unilateral block in one patient and extravasation of contrast medium in the other.

All patients with selective microsurgical removal of the polyp showed patent tubes on the control hysterosalpingography.

No pregnancy, however, has occurred during the follow-up period.

DISCUSSION

Resection of tubocornual polyps can be performed with microsurgical techniques without risk of blocking the tubes. Although no pregnancy occurred in eight patients with large bilateral tubocornual polyps the microsurgical technique may be a valuable adjuvant for treatment.

Analysis of the literature[1,5-9] on tubocornual polyps indicates that they are frequently associated with endometriosis, endometrial hyperplasia or polyps and uterine fibromyoma and may be part of a more generalized pathology of the genital tract. The treatment is therefore complex and may require a more sophisticated approach including hormonal and surgical. In our group of patients no hormonal treatment was given and in six patients additional pelvic surgery was performed for endometriosis (four patients) and uterine fibroma (two patients).

The question is still open as to whether tubocornual polyps with otherwise patent tubes must be treated. However, bilateral large polyps can be associated with long-standing primary subfertility and it is unlikely that large polyps will disintegrate with hormonal treatment[8,9].

References

1. Philipp, F. and Huber, H. (1939). Cause of endometriosis with a contribution on the pathology of the interstitial portion of the tube. *Zbl. Gynäk.*, **63**, 7
2. Lisa, J. R., Gioia, J. D. and Reehin, I. C. (1954). Observations on the interstitial portion of the fallopian tube. *Surg. Gynec. Obstet.*, **99**, 159–69
3. Zanesek, I. (1959). Die Salpingogramme bei der Endometrium hyperplasie. *Fartsch. Rontgenstr.*, **90**, 221–23
4. Ferström, I. and Lagerlof, B. (1964). Polyps in the intramural part of the fallopian tubes. A radiographic and clinical study. *J. Obstet. Gynaecol. Br. Commonw.*, **71**, 681–91
5. Bret, A. J. and Grepinet, J. (1967). Polypes endométriaux de la portion intramurale de la trompe. Leur rapport avec la stérilité et l'endometriose. *Sem. Hôp. Paris*, **43**, 183–92
6. Gaudefroy, M. and Empereur-Becissem, S. (1970). Les polypes endometriaux de la portion intramurale de la trompe. *Rev. Fr. Gynecol. Obstet.*, **65**, 571–8
7. Corette, L. (1977). La polypose de la portion intramurale de la trompe. Presented at the *Mémoire pour l'agrégation*, March, Lille
8. Gordts, S., Boeckx, W. and Brosens, I. (1983). Microsurgical resection of intramural tubal polyps. *Fertil. Steril.*, **40**, 258
9. Gordts, S., Boeckx, W., Vasquez, Gl. and Brosens, I. (1984). Microsurgical treatment of tubo-cornual polyps. In Phillips, J. (ed.) *Microsurgery in Gynecology II.* (In press)

Part V

Section 3
Clinical Results

45
Therapy and long-term results after different operative procedures for extrauterine pregnancy

M. LANGER, M. METKA, W. GRÜNBERGER and E. KUBISTA

The diagnosis of tubal pregnancy has undergone important changes in recent years: the introduction of new non-invasive methods like the LH/hCG test[1] or ultrasound equipment with high-dissolution capacity, and invasive methods like laparoscopy. Thus diagnosis of ectopic pregnancy has been made possible at a very early stage, sometimes even before the onset of clinical symptoms.

In patients after treatment for sterility or after disturbed pregnancy diagnostic measures are usually begun early. Consequently, tubal pregnancies found upon laparotomy often are small and show no clinical symptoms.

Since many of the patients in the departments of university hospitals have undergone treatment for sterility, the question as to the choice of surgical procedure plays an important role. Undoubtedly, total extirpation of the organ diminishes the chances for further pregnancies. Several authors, however, state that a conservative surgical procedure does not have a marked improvement on the fertility rate. Moreover, they suggest that it increases the danger of a recurring tubal pregnancy, not only on the side operated on, but also contralaterally[2,3]. Other authors are in favour of conservative procedures[4–6].

This chapter is designed to cast light on previously unclear therapeutic suggestions by way of the patient population examined at our department.

We compared 34 patients who were operated on conservatively (Table 1) with 38 patients undergoing radical operation. The findings on the contralateral fallopian tube were comparable in both groups. Conservative surgery either consisted in exprimation of the pregnancy through the ampullary os or in tubal resection with salpingostomy or sectio tubae.

Table 1 Operative procedures

Surgical procedure	*No. of patients*	*Contralateral fallopian tube*	
		Open	*Closed*
Conservative:			
Exprimation	15	4	1
Tubal resection with salpingostomy	11	9	0
Sectio tubae	8	1	2
Total	34	14	3
Radical (tubal extirpation)	38	15	10
Grand total	72	29	13

In all cases, we performed a salpingostomy, salpingolysis or adhesiolysis on the contralateral side if necessary. We were able to carry out a thorough follow-up examination in 41 of the 72 patients 1–5 years after surgery. Twenty-two of them had been operated on conservatively, 19 of them radically. Twenty-two of the 41 patients consented to a hysterosalpingography. It is self-evident that among these patients there were women who still wanted to become pregnant and for this reason they consented to a further investigation of their infertility.

Table 2 Follow-up results

Surgical procedure	*Follow-ups*	*Pregnancy*	*Ectopic pregnancy*
Conservative:			
Exprimation	12	5	2
Tubal resection with salpingostomy	7	2	2
Sectio tubae	3	0	0
Total	22	7	4
Radical (tubal extirpation)	19	2	0
Grand total	41	9	4

RESULTS

Table 2 shows that among the 22 women undergoing conservative operation there were seven intrauterine pregnancies, whereas among the 19 patients undergoing radical operation only two pregnancies occurred. It seems important to emphasize that five of the pregnancies were observed among the 12 patients who only had an exprimation of the tubal pregnancy. It may thus be concluded that the pregnancy rate was markedly higher in the group with conservative surgery. A repeated ectopic pregnancy occurred four times. All of these were in the group undergoing the conservative procedure; two of the four tubal pregnancies were located in the operated tube.

Twelve of the patients undergoing conservative operation underwent hysterosalpingography and have not yet become pregnant. The operated tube showed a normal X-ray in six cases, so that normal function may be concluded. In the radically operated group, four open and six closed tubes were reported (Table 3). In one individual case we could demonstrate a pregnancy through the operated fallopian tube, after extirpation of the contralateral side.

Table 3 Follow-up results after hysterosalpingography (HSG)

	HSG operated		*HSG contralateral*	
Surgical procedure	*Open*	*Closed*	*Open*	*Closed*
Exprimation	1	2	3	0
Tubal resection with salpingostomy	3	3	6	0
Sectio tubae	2	0	2	1
Tubal extirpation	0	10	4	6
Total	6	15	15	7

The following therapeutic procedure may be recommended for tubal pregnancies:

(1) Radical extirpation of the fallopian tube only in patients who do not plan to have any more children or whose tubal pregnancies would have an unfavourable location (interstitial), as well as in situations where the possibility of reconstruction of a functioning oviduct is impossible.

(2) In all other cases conservative procedure should be the method of choice, especially if the woman plans further pregnancies and if the contralateral adnexae finding excludes further conception.

(3) If an emergency situation arises, where the patient cannot give any statement about the operative procedure to be chosen, the conservative technique is to be applied for forensic reasons.

After conservative tubal surgery all patients must be informed about the risk of a repeated ectopic pregnancy and should contact their gynaecologist immediately after a menstrual period has been missed or a pregnancy suspected.

References

1. Grünberger, W., Leodolter, S. and Spona, J. (1978). The 'LH/HCG-test', a valuable aid in the diagnosis of tubal pregnancy. *Gynecol. Obstet. Invest.*, **9**, 150–5
2. Meirik, O. (1981). Ectopic pregnancy during 1961–1978 in Uppsala County, Sweden. *Acta Obstet. Gynecol. Scand.*, **60**, 545–8
3. Stolp, W. (1982). Extrauteringravidität. *Fortschr. Med.*, **100**, 754–9
4. Bruhat, M.A., Manhes, H., Mage, G. and Pouly, J.L. (1980). Treatment of ectopic pregnancy by means of laparoscopy. *Fertil. Steril.*, **33**, 411–14
5. Gomel, V. (1978). Salpingostomy by microsurgery. *Fertil. Steril.*, **29**, 380
6. Kitchin, J.D., Wein, R.M., Nunley, W.C., Thiagarajah, S. and Thornton, W.N. (1979). Ectopic pregnancy: current clinical trends. *Am. J. Obstet. Gynecol.*, **134**, 870–6

46
Emergency microsurgery

I. EIBSCHITZ, K. DE VRIES, M. HAKIM and M. SHARF

During the last 2 years we have used microsurgical techniques in 48 patients with gynaecological pelvic emergencies like ectopic pregnancies and ovarian cysts. In contrast to elective microsurgical procedures ('elective microsurgery') performed solely for existing mechanical infertility, we find it apt to describe this group as 'emergency microsurgery' group, in which microsurgical techniques are used because of possible desire for children in the future.

The characteristics of our 'emergency microsurgery' group are shown in Table 1. Comparing our 'emergency microsurgery' group with the 'elective microsurgery' group we found it possible to attribute certain characteristics to both (Table 2). It became clear that results from 'emergency microsurgery' operations cannot be compared as to pregnancies achieved, since some of the

Table 1 Characteristics of 'emergency microsurgery' group

No. of cases	*Diagnosis*	*Type of 'emergency microsurgery'*
24	Tubal pregnancy	Milking out (1), dorsal salpingotomy (13), partial salpingectomy (6) and microsurgical salpingectomy (4)
2	Ovarian pregnancy	Ovarian wedge resection[1]
1	Rudimentary horn pregnancy	Rudimentary horn resection
15	Ovarian cyst	Cystectomy
2	Torsion of adnexa	Adnexectomy
4	Torsion of cyst	Cystectomy

patients were schoolgirls and some of the adults were using contraceptives after the operations. Nevertheless, microsurgical techniques were used in all these cases so as to prevent the possibility of mechanical infertility in the future.

Table 2 Characteristics of both groups of patients undergoing microsurgery

Characteristic	*'Emergency microsurgery'*	*Elective microsurgery*
Age of patients	Childhood – end of fertility age	Only fertility age
Timing of operation	Night or day, according to urgency	Only day, proliferative phase
Antibiotics	Only intra- or postoperative	Pre-, intra- and postoperative
Corticosteroids	Not given	Given in most cases
Pregnancy desire	Mostly not existing at time of operation	Always existing at time of operation
No. of procedures per operation	Average: 1.3	Average: 2.3
Results of operation	Not comparable (as to pregnancies achieved)	Comparable (as to pregnancies achieved)
Extent of peritoneal damage	Sometimes known before the operation	Always known before operation

In the emergency group, preoperative antibiotics could not be administered as in the elective group, from the evening before the operation, since most cases had to be operated upon shortly after their arrival. Corticosteroids were not given in 'emergency microsurgery' with haemorrhage and oedema, as they were in 'elective microsurgery'. The number of different procedures performed during one single operation (for example, dorsal salpingotomy and also ovarian cystectomy) was significantly lower in the 'emergency mirosurgery group, on average 1.3 compared with 2.3 in the 'elective microsurgery' group. This is due to focal pathology in the emergency group and the need for the operator to do only the essential procedure during emergency operations.

The concept of emergency microsurgery seems important to us and should be considered in all cases of urgent pelvic, including non-gynaecological surgery like appendicectomy, in all female patients from infancy until the end of the reproductive age, in view of the importance of preventing future mechanical infertility, which might be called 'iatrogenic infertility' if microsurgical technique were not used[2].

References

1. de Vries, K., Shapiro, I., Degani, S., Levitan, Z., Mitrani, A. and Sharf, M. (1983). Ovarian pregnancy in association with an intrauterine device. *Int. J. Gynaecol. Obstet.*, **21**, 65
2. Winston, R. M. L. (1980). Microsurgery in female infertility. In Crosignani and Rubin (eds.) *Atraumatic Conservative Pelvic Surgery*. p. 121 (New York: Academic Press; Grune and Stratton)

47
Pelvic microsurgery in an Irish context

M. R. N. DARLING

INTRODUCTION

In March 1982 I introduced the operating microscope to the Rotunda Hospital, Dublin, and in this chapter I hope to explain my first year's experience. Prior to 1982 I had gained 3½ years' experience in pelvic microsurgery at Hammersmith Hospital, London, with Robert Winston and Raoul Magara.

During the year under review 190 laparoscopies were performed for the evaluation of female infertility problems. 51 patients were found to have anatomical distortion but seven of these patients were unsuitable for microsurgical operative techniques due to gross structural damage.

A total of 44 operations was performed using the Wild M.650 Operating Microscope. Only two patients were referred for the reversal of sterilization operation – aged 44 and 37 years, respectively. Reversal was achieved in both cases with good technical results but neither patient has become pregnant. At least one of these patients is, to my best knowledge, not keen to conceive and the reversal procedure was, in retrospect, I believe, performed mainly to allay a guilt complex resulting from the initial operation. Female sterilization is an uncommon procedure in Ireland.

The remaining 42 ladies received tubal surgery with magnification using the microsurgical approach. Twenty-seven patients came through our own Infertility Clinic, 15 being referred to me by other gynaecologists. The average age was 30.4 years and 25 complained of primary infertility, 10 had at least one previous live child, five had had a previous ectopic pregnancy and two a previous abortion as their only obstetric history.

Thirty-two of the 42 patients had had some previous pelvic interference –

including appendicectomy, ovarian cystectomy, ectopic pregnancy and previous infertility surgery for endometriosis or structural problems. All patients had preoperative laparoscopies and full infertility work-ups. At laparotomy the major cause of pelvic damage, as assessed by me, was infection in 24 patients (57%), endometriosis in nine, previous surgery in five and congenital anomalies in four.

SURGERY

The surgery performed was salpingostomy in 13 patients, isthmic-cornual anastomosis in nine and adhesiolysis in 20. (Under the term adhesiolysis I include salpingolysis, ovariolysis, ovarian cystectomy, myomectomy and a combination of these.)

Follow-up ranges from 3 to 15 months and 16 patients are at present receiving other concomitant therapy (mainly ovarian stimulation). For 35% of patients current follow-up is less than 6 months.

RESULTS

There were five cases of intrauterine pregnancy and two cases of ectopic pregnancy. Thus seven patients have become pregnant; unfortunately two of these were ectopic tubal pregnancies. Both these patients had adhesiolysis type operations and one had had a previous salpingectomy for ectopic pregnancy on the other side. Five ongoing intrauterine pregnancies (12%) of total operations) include two from the salpingostomy group, two who had isthmic-cornual anastomosis and one who had salpingo-oopholysis.

The purpose of this chapter is to report that, even in Ireland, post-inflammatory damage is a major contributor to Ireland's subfertility problem.

48
Microsurgical restoration of tuboperitoneal infertility in 125 women

S. SARRIS, A. COMNINOS and K. MAVRELOS

INTRODUCTION

Operative procedures to reconstruct occluded tubes and those involved with significant adhesions have been described for more than a century but were never satisfactory until recently when microsurgical techniques were introduced[1].

Although microsurgery versus macrosurgery is still a controversial issue[2,3], published reports[4-7] from many centres show that microsurgical techniques improve the success rate with tuboplasty and could represent a significant step forward in infertility surgery.

In this chapter we report our results of various types of microsurgical salpingoplasty performed on 125 patients at Marika Eliadi Maternity Hospital in Athens.

MATERIALS AND METHODS

From September 1978 to December 1982, 125 patients between 21 and 39 years of age (mean 27 years) underwent microsurgical tuboplasty.

Of the 125 patients, 39 complained of primary infertility and 86 of secondary infertility. The outcome of last pregnancy in the latter were 12 miscarriages, 68 induced abortions and six ectopic pregnancies. Twenty-seven out of the 125 patients had previous laparotomy for reasons other than infertility.

All patients received a complete infertility evaluation and other causes of infertility were excluded. Hysterosalpingography and laparoscopy were utilized to evaluate the tubal status prior to surgery. Patients who were found to have endometriosis at laparoscopy were excluded from this study.

As an operating microscope we employed the Olympus MTX colposcope with oculars 10 × magnification.

During the operation all patients received 750 mg Zinacef, 1 fl Flagyl (metronidazole) and 500 mg hydrocortisone succinate intravenously. The antibiotics were given intravenously through the second day and then by mouth through the 15th postoperative day. Dexamethasone 10 mg by mouth was started from the first postoperative day, gradually discontinued through the 10th postoperative day. An 8–0 Prolene suture was used for tubal reconstruction and restoration of damaged peritoneum.

The cul-de-sac was loosely packed with tapes moistened with solution of normal saline and heparin 5000 IU^{-1}. Irrigation with solution of normal saline and heparin rather than sponging was used to keep the operative field clean. Dissection was made with unipolar electrosurgery and haemostasis was achieved by bipolar microsurgical forceps. At the completion of tuboplasty and prior to closing the peritoneum, the pelvic cavity was lavaged with a solution of normal saline and heparin and after that 1.5 g of hydrocortisone succinate was left inside.

Hydrotubation was not performed pre- or postoperatively but only during the operation in those patients who underwent salpingoneostomy. Our patients were divided into four groups according to the type of microsurgical operation. The first group refers to bilateral terminal salpingostomy that was performed in 65 cases. The dimple in the blocked end was sometimes clear and was sometimes identified by distention of the tube with diluted methylene blue injected through the fundus of the uterus into the cavity.

The initial tubal incision was made with the electrical microneedle. Consequently the mucosa was cuffed back and sutured to the tubal serosa with an 8/0 Prolene suture.

The second group consisted of 33 patients undergoing fimbrioplasty. Most of these cases underwent deagglutination. The third group comprised five patients in whom isthmic–isthmic anastomosis was performed and four in whom the blockage was postabortal while the remaining patient was sterilized during her second caesarean section.

The fourth group consisted of 22 patients undergoing combined operations. These combined operations included different operations on right and left tubes. Since adhesion formation of various degrees was found salpingolysis was performed, at the same time, in all patients.

RESULTS

Table 1 presents the results of microsurgical tuboplasty in 125 patients with a minimum of 6 months postoperative follow-up. From the 85 patients who underwent salpingostomy 22 (34%) became pregnant in a total of 24 pregnancies. The procedure of fimbrioplasty was used to treat 33 patients, 18 (54%) of whom became pregnant. In the anastomosis group of five patients three (60%) conceived. Combined operations were performed in 22 patients, nine (41%) of whom became pregnant.

Table 1 Results of microsurgical tuboplasty in 125 patients; 6 months minimum postoperative follow-up

Operation	*No. of patients*		*No. of pregnancies*
	Operated	*Pregnant*	
Salpingostomy (terminal)	65	22 (34%)	24
Fimbrioplasty	33	18 (54%)	20
Anastomosis	5	3 (60%)	3
Combinations	22	9 (41%)	13
Total	125	52 (41.6%)	60

The outcome of the pregnancies is given in Table 2. From the 24 pregnancies of the salpingostomy group, nine ended in full-term delivery, three are in progress, six miscarried and six (25%) were ectopic. The total fetal wastage was 50%.

Table 2 Outcome of 60 pregnancies in 52 patients who conceived after microsurgical tuboplasty

Operation	*No. of pregnancies*	*No. of deliveries*	*No. in progress*	*No. of miscarriages*	*No. ectopic*	*Fetal wastage (%)*
Salpingostomy	24	9	3	6	6 (25%)	50
Fimbrioplasty	20	9	3	5	3 (15%)	40
Anastomosis	3	3	–	–	–	0
Combinations	13	5	2	6	–	46
Total	60	26	8	17	9	45

From the 20 pregnancies of the fimbrioplasty group, nine ended in full-term delivery, three are presently well, five miscarried and three (15%) were ectopic.

The three pregnancies after isthmic–isthmic anastomosis went to term. From the 13 pregnancies in the combined operations group five went to term, two are in progress and six aborted.

References

1. Swolin, K. (1967). Fifty fertility operations: literature and methods. *Acta Obstet. Gynecol. Scand.*, **46**, 234
2. Jones. H. W. and Rock, J. A. (1976). On the reanastomosis of the fallopian tubes after surgical sterilization. *Fertil. Steril.*, **29**, 702
3. Gomel, V. (1977). Tubal reanastomosis by microsurgery. *Fertil. Steril.*, **28**, 59
4. Swolin, K. (1975). Electromicrosurgery and salpingoneostomy: long term results. *Am. J. Obstet. Gynecol.*, **121**, 418
5. Diamond, E. (1979). Lysis of postoperative pelvic adhesions in infertility. *Fertil. Steril.*, **31**, 287
6. Winston, R. M. L. (1977). Microsurgical tubocornual anastomosis for reversal of sterilization. *Lancet*, **1**, 284
7. Fayez, J. A. and Suliman, O. S. (1982). Infertility surgery of the oviduct: comparison between macrosurgery and microsurgery. *Fertil. Steril.*, **37**, 73

Part VI

Uterus and Vagina

49
Hysteroscopy in infertility

J. KAVVOS, S. SARRIS and A. COMNINOS

Despite the fact that the first hysteroscope was made in 1865 and the first gynaecological use of the instrument was reported in 1869, hysteroscopy is not widely used as a diagnostic and therapeutic method.

The revolution in the technology of endoscopy in the 1970s did not positively affect hysteroscopy as it did laparoscopy, and gynaecologists hesitate to adapt the method because of technical difficulties.

This chapter aims to present our experience in the use of hysteroscopy in cases of infertility, perhaps to stimulate more colleagues in its use.

MATERIALS AND METHOD

The hysteroscope used was the Storz model which consists of a rigid, 4 mm, 30 degree telescope and a 7 mm sheath and can accommodate a flexible instrument (scissors, biopsy forceps or palpator). The main light source used was the Storz 559 TTL which facilitates photographic documentation. Dextran 6% in normal saline under manually maintained positive pressure was used to distend the uterus.

All hysteroscopies were performed in the operating theatre, under general anaesthesia, with the patient in the lithotomy position. The preparation of the vagina with antiseptics was followed by catheterization of the bladder and careful dilatation of the cervix to Hegar No 7. The hysteroscope was advanced into the cervical canal under direct vision.

31 infertile patients underwent hysteroscopy in the first 12 months of application of the method in our unit.

The indications for hysteroscopy included:

Abnormal hysterogram (adhesions?), 18 patients.
Prolonged, unexplained infertility, seven patients.
Intrauterine adhesions, two patients.
Pregnancy wastage, one patient.
Secondary amenorrhoea, one patient.
Intracervical adhesions, one patient.
Previous dilatation and currettage (allergic to urographin for hysterogram), one patient.

Hysteroscopy was done either as a single procedure or combined with others, as follows.

In six cases the operation was hysteroscopy only. In seven cases hysteroscopy was followed by dilatation and curettage. In 13 cases hysteroscopy was combined with laparoscopy and in five cases hysteroscopy was combined with laparoscopy and dilatation and curettage.

An apparent cause of infertility was found intra-abdominally in 12 out of the 18 laparoscoped patients. In the 13 cases of hysteroscopy which were not combined with laparoscopy, hysteroscopy was performed during the early proliferative part of the cycle, whereas in the other 18 cases hysteroscopy was done during the secretory phase.

In cases that required lysis of intrauterine adhesions, an IUCD was placed in the uterus and antibiotics, betamethasone and oestrogens were administered systematically for 1 week after the operation to prevent recurrence of adhesions.

RESULTS

In 24 cases a normal cervical canal was seen. In the remaining seven intracervical adhesions of various severity were diagnosed.

In 26 cases the internal cervical os was judged as competent, while in five cases cervical incompetence was diagnosed.

The main hysteroscopic findings were as follows:

Intrauterine adhesions, 14 patients. (In five of these intracervical adhesions coexisted.)
Intrauterine polyp(s), six patients.
Intracervical adhesions only, two patients.
Submucosal fibroids, two patients.
Products of pregnancy, one patient.
Adenomatous hyperplasia, one patient.

In four cases no abnormality was seen, while in another patient we failed to visualize the uterine cavity because of the presence of blood due to the laparoscopic manipulation of the uterus before the hysteroscopy (Figures 1–5).

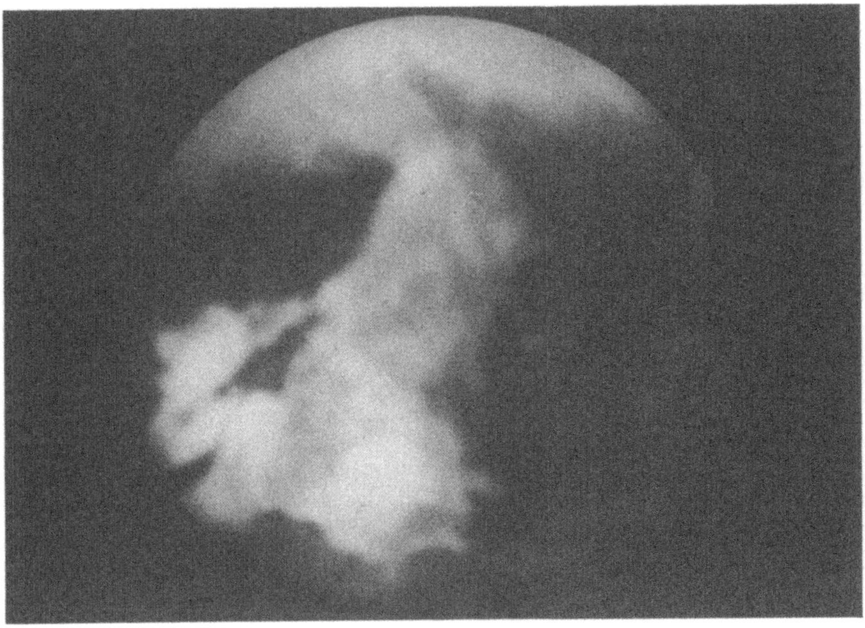

Figure 1 Endometrial polyp

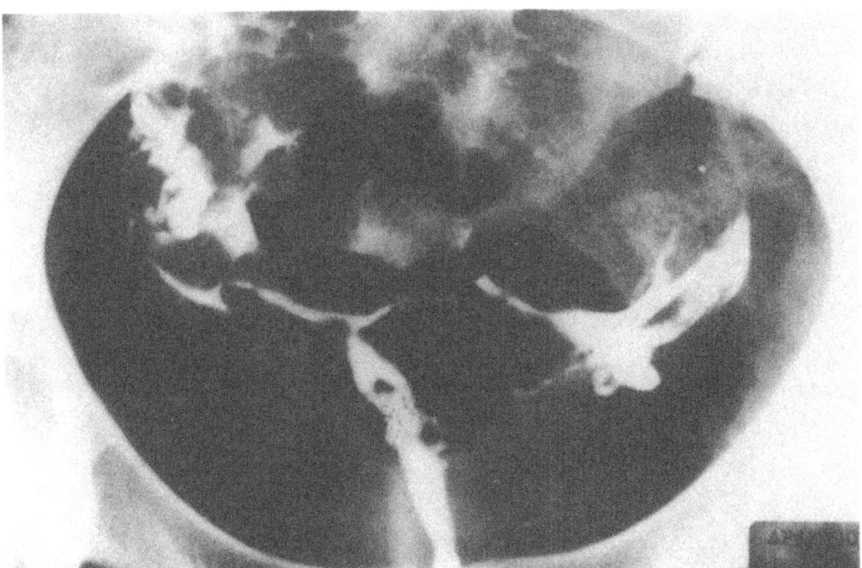

Figure 2 Endometrial adhesions

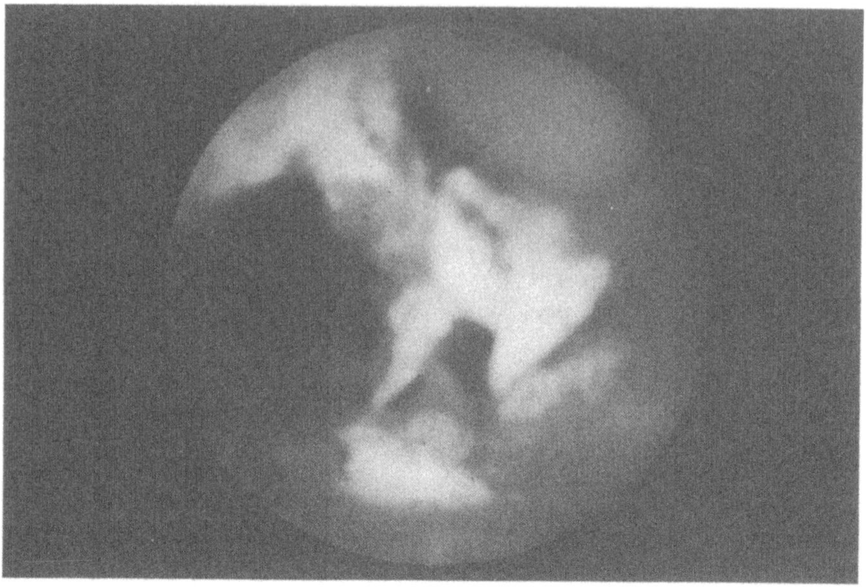

Figures 3 and 4 Endometrial adhesions; same patient as in Figure 2

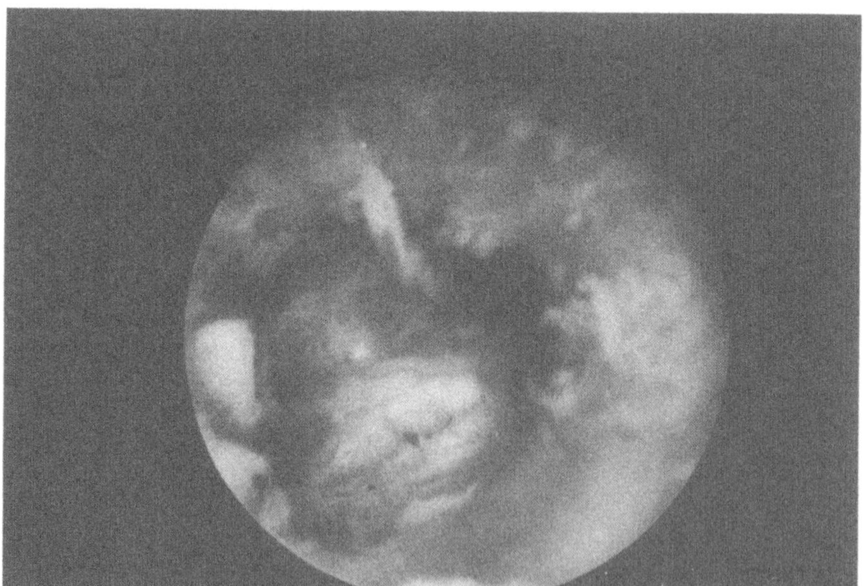

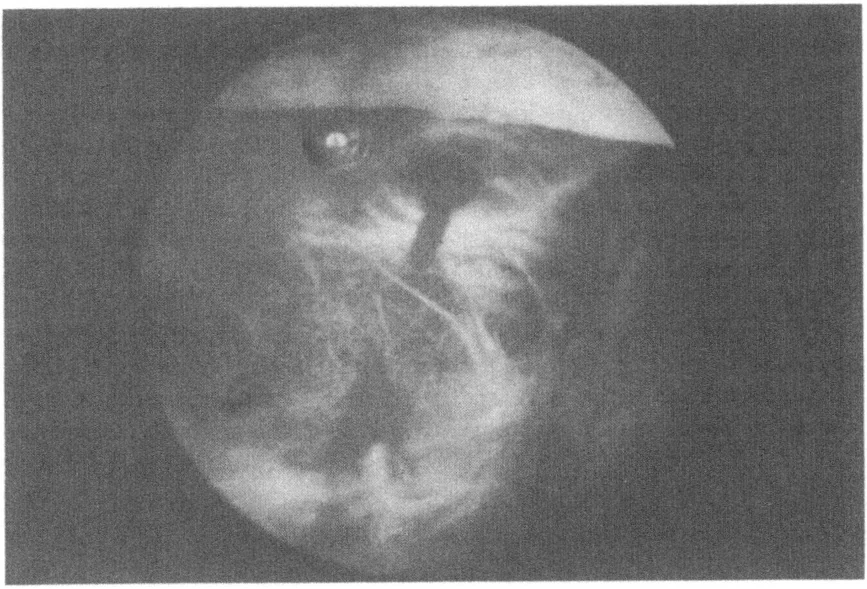

Figure 5 Partial perforation of uterine wall, with slight bleeding

In cases with intrauterine and intracervical adhesions hysteroscopic separation was performed with the use of flexible miniature scissors. In cases of endometrial polyps and abnormal endometrium a curettage was performed.

Two perforations of the uterus occurred during the early days of application of the method. Both occurred in cases with diffuse intrauterine adhesions with blockage of the uterine cavity. No laparotomy was required as the bleeding was laparoscopically classified as minimal. In two-thirds of our patients who were also laparoscoped there was an absolute tubo-ovarian cause of infertility.

Four of our patients became pregnant following the separation of endometrial adhesions and two of them have already had their babies at term. Another pregnancy was achieved after the removal of a big endometrial polyp and is near term now. A sixth pregnancy, in a case where no abnormality was seen during hysteroscopy, ended in a spontaneous abortion.

DISCUSSION

No difficulty was encountered during hysteroscopy in inspecting the cervical canal and the internal os, while considerable difficulty prevented us from inspecting the tubal ostium in some patients who were hysteroscoped during the secretory phase of the cycle.

A similar difficulty was encountered in patients with adenomatous hyperplasia, where in some instances large endometrial folds were taken as polyps.

The separation of intrauterine adhesions became easier and more effective as our experience increased. Progressively we were able to separate extensive rigid adhesions without difficulty.

The reported four pregnancies were achieved after separation of moderately extensive uterine adhesions while the two perforations occurred in cases with extremely extensive and rigid adhesions with complete blockage of the uterine cavity.

The number of our patients is too small for precise statistical conclusions. However, we feel that the hysteroscope is a valuable tool in the investigation, and in some cases in the treatment, of infertility and therefore hysteroscopy should be used more widely by physicians dealing with problems of infertility.

50
Treatment of intrauterine adhesions

D. NAVOT, E. J. MARGALIOTH, S. MOR-JOSEFF and J. G. SCHENKER

Partial or complete obliteration of the uterine cavity by adherence of the uterine walls, leading to menstrual abnormalities (usually amenorrhoea or hypomenorrhoea), infertility and habitual abortion, has been termed Asherman's syndrome or intrauterine adhesions (IUA).

After Asherman's repeated publications since 1948, the syndrome has acquired world-wide attention. Asherman was the first to point out the frequency of its appearance, and he described in detail the aetiology, symptoms and presented a roentgenological picture.

Diagnosis of IUA is based on a high index of suspicion and alertness to the existence of a number of predisposing factors like the gravid uterus, post-abortal and post-partum infections and missed abortions. IUA may also be caused by trauma and genital tuberculosis.

Over the last decade our department has been involved in clinical and experimental studies concerning intrauterine adhesions. 178 patients with IUA were diagnosed during the last decade in our department. The present report deals with the diagnosis and treatment of the specific cause of infertility.

DIAGNOSIS

Symptoms may vary according to the aetiology and the extent of IUA. On the one end of the spectrum it may present as an accidental finding without any clinical symptoms, and at the extreme end of the spectrum as IUA with intrauterine fibrosis or uterine atresia resulting in amenorrhoea. Symptoms, therefore, vary according to the extent of the disease but are always within two categories: infertility and menstrual disorders.

The category of infertility includes sterility, repeated and habitual abortion, and complications of late pregnancy such as premature labour, placenta praevia, and placenta accreta. The classic menstrual disorders are amenorrhoea and hypomenorrhoea, but dysmenorrhoea and menometorrhagia are also occasionally present.

Table 1 details the presenting symptoms in our patients. Diagnosis and location of IUA are based essentially on hysterography, which must be performed with a short cannula. The filling defects that have been ascribed to IUA are characterized by their irregularity, their angulated form, with very sharp contours, and their homogeneous opacity.

Table 1 Symptoms* of 178 patients with IUA

Symptoms	*No.*	*%*
Sterility	120	34
Hypomenorrhoea	83	23
Recurrent abortions	58	16
Normal menses	56	16
Amenorrhoea	39	11

* In cases where more than one symptom is noted, all are included.

TREATMENT AND PROGNOSIS

The treatment of IUA is a controversial subject. With a lasting cure in mind, treatment consists of removing the adhesions surgically and, at the same time, preventing formation of new ones.

Surgical removal of adhesions may be attempted via the vaginal route or abdominal hysterotomy, and by 'blind' curettage or through a hysteroscope. It is not settled whether blunt dissection or sharp severance is the more effective method. For the prevention of recurrence insertion of an intrauterine device (IUD) has been advocated[2]. An inflated Foley catheter may serve the same purpose[3]. Post-adhesiolysis antibiotics, steroids and oestrogen administration have been tried.

During the last decade we have utilized a special protocol for treatment of IUA. Of 178 patients, 153 were treated as follows:

(1) Lysis of adhesions by dilatation and curettage per vaginum in 137 patients and via hysterotomy in 16 patients.
(2) Immediate insertion of Y-shaped IUD for 4–8 weeks.
(3) Conjugated oestrogen 1.25 mg daily for 1 month.

Our results are summarized in Table 2.

Table 2 Menstruation and fertility in 153 women with IUA

Disorder	Treatment	No. of cases	Menstruation			Fertility		
			Normal menses	Hypomenorrhoea	Temporary menses only	Conceived	Abortion	Delivered
Intrauterine adhesions	D&C only	22	14 (64%)	8		16 (73%)	5	11
	D&C+Lippes IUD +conjugated oestrogens	26	20 (77%)	6		19 (73%)	6	13
	D&C+Y-shaped IUD +conjugated oestrogens	49	44 (90%)	5		41 (84%)	8	33
Cervical adhesions	D&C+Y-shaped IUD +conjugated oestrogens	40	38 (95%)	2		35 (87%)	3	32
Total		137	116 (85%)	21		111 (81%)		89
Total atresia	Through hysterotomy	4	1		3	0		
Genital tuberculosis	D&C+IUD	12	1		9	0		

D&C=Dilatation and curettage.

Normal menses were re-established in 116 (85%) patients out of the 137 who were treated vaginally. Of these 111 patients conceived, and 89 (80%) delivered a living child. Only 16 (14%) women had a complicated delivery; nine had premature deliveries; seven sustained post-partum bleeding and one suffered from placenta accreta. Lysis of adhesions through hysterotomy in treatment of complete obliteration of uterine cavity was disappointing. Treatment of adhesions associated with tuberculosis was a total failure with regard to pregnancy.

The universal incidence of intrauterine adhesions, or Asherman's syndrome, is steadily increasing. The syndrome is expressed mainly by infertility and menstrual disorders. Pregnancy, when achieved, may be complicated by premature labour, placenta praevia and placenta accreta. Amenorrhoea and hypomenorrhoea are the classic menstrual disorders. It is stressed that whenever these symptoms are manifest subsequent to uterine trauma, the existence of intrauterine adhesions should be strongly suspected. Although the diagnostic tool in common use is hysterography, for accurate diagnosis application of hysteroscopy is advocated. Preferred treatment is curettage followed by immediate insertion of an IUD, combined with a course of oestrogens. Present fertility results with these methods still merit improvement.

References

1. Toaff, R. and Ballas, S. (1978). Traumatic hypomenorrhoea-amenorrhea (Asherman's syndrome). *Fertil. Steril.*, **30**, 379
2. Jewelewicz, R., Khalaf, S., Neuwirth, R.S. and Vande Wiele, R.L. (1976). Obstetric complications after treatment of intrauterine synechiae (Asherman's syndrome). *Obstet. Gynecol.*, **47**, 701
3. Comninos, A.C. and Zourlas, P.A. (1969). Treatment of uterine adhesions (Asherman's syndrome). *Am. J. Obstet. Gynecol.*, **105**, 862

51
The place of metroplasty in the management of congenital uterine malformation

P. R. BOWMAN, N. M. DUIGNAN and A. T. GREENE

Congenital uterine malformation has long been recognized as a cause of recurrent pregnancy failures and also of dysmenorrhoea. Treatment has changed over the years from initially one of expectant management through the era of cervical cerclage to most recently, surgical correction of the uterine defect, as recommended by Strassman[1].

We wish to report the circumstances of, and the results obtained in nine patients who underwent Strassman's metroplasty in the Coombe Lying-In Hospital, Dublin.

Between 1974 and 1980, nine patients were identified as having bicornuate uteri. Seven of these presented with recurrent pregnancy failures, one with primary infertility and one with severe dysmenorrhoea.

In the previously pregnant group two women gave a history of three and six first-trimester abortions respectively, whilst in the remaining five cases the more usual pattern of mid-trimester pregnancy loss was observed (Table 1).

Table 1 Previous history in patients with bicornuate uteri, 1974–1980

Case no.	
1	Abortions at 18, 18 and 22 weeks
2	Premature labour at 28, 29 and 28 weeks (neonatal death × 3)
3	Abortions at 13, 6, 13, 9, 9 and 14 weeks
4	Abortions at 12, 6 and 12 weeks
5	Abortions at 24 and 22 weeks
6	Abortions at 18, 21 and 17 weeks
7	Abortions at 16, 17 and 21 weeks

The uterine abnormality was diagnosed following two abortions in one patient, after three abortions in each of four patients and in one woman after her third neonatal death. A further patient did not present until after her sixth abortion. Maternal age at diagnosis varied between 20 and 35 years.

In another case the uterine abnormality was noted during routine infertility investigations. Interestingly, in addition this lady had polycystic ovarian disease. Along with bilateral ovarian wedge resection, she also underwent a standardized Strassman's metroplasty.

Having been extensively investigated and treated at other hospitals over a period of 3 years, a 17-year-old schoolgirl was referred to the Coombe Hospital for further assessment of incapacitating dysmenorrhoea. Her history was one of frequent absences from school during menstruation because of recurrent episodes of severe colicky lower abdominal pain. Despite a planned 'cold' appendicectomy, examination under anaesthesia with dilatation of the cervix and anovulant therapy her symptoms had persisted. At laparoscopy a bicornuate uterus was noted and she too underwent a Strassman's procedure.

METHODS

The nine metroplàsties were performed by each of the three authors, in a standardized fashion. Uterine tissue adjacent to the defect was excised and the myometrium reconstituted in three layers to form a single endometrial cavity. Scrupulous attention was paid to good haemostasis in an attempt to minimize omental adhesion formation. Prophylactic antibiotic therapy was not prescribed. All the patients were discharged from hospital within 12 days of their surgery.

RESULTS

The patient with primary infertility failed to ovulate subsequently, despite appropriate therapy. The schoolgirl with dysmenorrhoea was dramatically cured of her symptoms. She was followed up for a period of a year without recurrence of her complaint and without further interruption to her schooling. To quote her highly appreciative mother, 'the domestic situation has been totally transformed'.

In the seven patients with recurrent abortion, spontaneous conceptions occurred at 5, 6, 8, 10 and 12 months respectively. Clomiphene was necessary to induce ovulation in two women whose conceptions occurred at 1 year and 2 years respectively following surgery (Table 2).

In all cases the immediate post-surgery conception was successful. Five patients were delivered by elective caesarean section, performed between the 38th and 39th week. In two women the membranes ruptured spontaneously at

Table 2 Surgery–conception interval in patients with bicornuate uteri, 1974–1980

Case no.		*Interval* (months)
1	Spontaneous pregnancy	6
2	Clomiphene-induced pregnancy	12
3	Spontaneous pregnancy	5
4	Spontaneous pregnancy	10
5	Spontaneous pregnancy	12
6	Spontaneous pregnancy	8
7	Clomiphene-induced pregnancy	24

37 weeks and in each instance an emergency section was carried out. With one exception the pregnancies were totally uncomplicated. One woman suffered from intermittent attacks of abdominal pain from 26 weeks until delivery for which no cause could be found.

In each case the baby was healthy at birth. There were no congenital abnormalities and birth weights varied between 2.68 and 3.91 kg (Table 3).

Table 3 Infants born to patients with bicornuate uteri, 1974–1980

Case no.	*Gestation* (weeks)	*Weight* (kg)
1	37	2.68
2	38	3.56
3	39	2.74
4	38	3.91
5	37	3.03
6	39	3.45
7	38	3.40

Despite the extensive uterine surgery, adhesion formation was noted in only one patient subsequently and this was the only case in which it was necessary to perform a classical section. This variation was decided upon at operation, when problems mobilizing the bladder were encountered. Scar dehiscence did not occur, in fact without exception myometrial thickness was a notable feature.

Four patients embarked on further pregnancies following their first post-metroplasty pregnancy and in one case a third pregnancy was conceived. With one exception these pregnancies also yielded healthy infants. Unfortunately one baby died *in utero* at 25 weeks from a cord complication which was obviously unrelated to the previous surgery (Table 4).

In summary, therefore, out of nine women who underwent metroplasty, eight healthy babies were born to seven women who had previously lost 23

Table 4 Further pregnancies in patients with bicornuate uteri, 1974–1980

Case no.	*Year*	*Pregnancy*
1	1980	SROM @ 37 weeks emergency CS. Male, 2.68 kg A/W
	1982	Abruptio @ 34 weeks emergency CS. Male, 2.46 kg A/W
3	1976	Elective CS 39 weeks. Female, 2.74 kg A/W
	1976	Elective CS 39 weeks. Female, 2.75 kg A/W
	1982	Elective CS 38 weeks. Male, 3.00 kg A/W
4	1981	Elective CS 39 weeks. Male, 3.91 kg A/W
	1983	Elective CS 38 weeks. Male, 3.94 kg A/W
6	1980	Elective CS (classical) 39 weeks. Male, 3.45 kg A/W
	1981	IUD 25 weeks aborted at 31 weeks, cord strictures

CS = Caesarean section; A/W = alive and well; IUD = intrauterine death.

pregnancies due directly to a congenital uterine defect. There was one intrauterine death which was unavoidable.

A young schoolgirl was totally cured of her distressing dysmenorrhoea with restoration of a normal schooling pattern.

In one instance surgery conferred no benefit as the coexisting ovarian disease proved refractory to all modes of therapy (Table 5).

Table 5 Summary of results in patients with bicornuate uteri, 1974–1980

Symptoms	*Procedure*	*Results*
23 pregnancy failures	Metroplasty × 7	9 healthy infants
Severe disruptive dysmenorrhoea	Metroplasty	Total relief
Primary infertility	Metroplasty	No benefit

DISCUSSION

These results clearly demonstrate the value of energetic investigation of the recurrent aborter and of atypical dysmenorrhoea. Of particular interest are the two patients whose congenital uterine defect was associated with first-trimester pregnancy loss, a condition for which one might not readily consider hysterosalpingography in its assessment. Uterine malformation should also be considered in all cases of atypical dysmenorrhoea, as the above patient clearly demonstrates, since the benefits of surgery can be so worthwhile. Lastly as the two patients who required clomiphene illustrate, pregnancy may be delayed following surgery and additional therapy may be required before achieving a successful outcome.

References

1. Strassman, E.D. (1961). Operations for double uterus and endometrial atresia. *Clin. Obstet. Gynaecol.*, **4**, 240–55

52
Psychosexual consequences of Vecchietti's operation in Rockitansky–Küster–Hauser syndrome

P. RISS, K. SCHIEDER, A. M. ROGAN and H. JANISCH

The large number of different operations proposed for formation of a neovagina in congenital or acquired absence of the vagina shows that an operation satisfactory in all respects is still missing. In recent years Vecchietti's operation has attracted attention. The ideal operation should fulfil different criteria: the operation should be technically simple and without major complications, other organ systems should not be involved, intercourse should be possible soon after the operation, follow-up care should be simple and there should be no disagreeable vaginal discharge.

VECCHIETTI'S OPERATION

Vecchietti's operation is based on the method described by Frank[1] in which a new vagina is created by exerting pressure on the region between the urethral orifice and the anus. In Vecchietti's operation the neovagina is formed not by pressure from the perineum but by traction from the small pelvis. This is achieved by placing a small plastic olive on the perineum, and by pulling the olive inwards by two threads. The threads are placed through the abdominal wall after a Pfannenstiel laparotomy and fixed to a spring apparatus to ensure adequate traction. Traction is increased every other day; after approximately 10 days the olive is removed. At this time the neovagina has reached a length of about 9 cm[2,3].

PATIENTS AND RESULTS

Vecchietti's operation was performed in eight patients with Rockitansky-Küster-Hauser syndrome, in one patient with testicular feminization, and in one patient with vaginal occlusion after hysterectomy and post-operative radiotherapy because of endometrial cancer. In all patients there was at least a small vaginal pouch; twice we found abnormalities of the kidneys (one aplasia, one pelvic kidney) which emphasizes the need to do pre-operative intravenous pyelograms.

The olive was removed between the 7th and 12th postoperative day. At this time the definitive length of the neovagina was reached but the diameter of the neovagina was still insufficient and had to be gradually increased by use of vaginal dilators. On discharge from the hospital, the neovagina was wide enough to admit two fingers in six out of 10 patients. However, in the patient with occlusion of the vagina after radiotherapy it was not possible to keep the neovagina open; on follow-up 13 months postoperatively the neovagina was again completely occluded and intercourse was not possible; the patient suffered from depression and was habitually taking alcohol. In hindsight, we would say that this patient was not a suitable candidate for a Vecchietti operation. Preoperatively seven out of nine patients had stable partnerships and at least some sexual experience. Oral or anal sexual activity was reported by three and two women, respectively. It is interesting to note that half of the patients reported orgasm, though this is of course difficult to verify.

On follow-up 2–20 months postoperatively the majority of patients had satisfactory results (Table 1). In two women the length of the neovagina was only 5 cm, the epithelium was complete in all cases and not distinguishable from normal vaginal epithelium. Patient 9 had no stable sexual partner 5 months after the operation and had no possibility of regular sexual intercourse.

More important than the morphological result, however, is whether the patient is satisfied and whether the neovagina permits normal and gratifying intercourse. The majority of our patients were satisfied and believed that their sexual partner also found intercourse satisfactory. In two women there was a change in sexual partners after the operation. No patient complained of dyspareunia, and all patients reported orgasm. Since intercourse was possible in all patients, and since seven out of eight patients and their partners found intercourse satisfactory one would conclude that the length of the neovagina is not the most important factor.

COMMENT

Vecchietti's operation for formation of a neovagina is technically simple and easily supported by the patient. Other advantages of the operation include

Table 1 Neovagina on follow-up

	Neovagina					
Patient	*Follow-up* (months)	*Length* (cm)	*Diameter* (fingers)	*Epithelium*	*Vaginal discharge*	*Vaginal dilator*
1	20	9	Two	+	0	0
2	20	8	Two	+	(+)	0
3	16	8	Two	+	(+)	0
5	9	9	Two	(+)	(+)	At night
6	9	5	Two	+	0	0
7	5	8	Two	+	0	At night
8	Patient not available for follow-up					
9	5	5	Two	(+)	+	Day and night
10	2	10	Two	+	0	At night

the absence of significant vaginal discharge and the possibility of early intercourse. We emphasized manual exploration of the neovagina by the patient and her partner, and recommended first attempts at intercourse about 3 weeks after the operation. In our experience patients of slightly advanced age and with sufficient preoperative sexual experience did better postoperatively: these patients were able to adjust much more easily to the neovagina psychologically and were able to explore fully the possibilities offered by the neovagina together with their partners.

Any operation for formation of a neovagina is only one step in the treatment of vaginal aplasia. In fact many investigators have stressed that the type of procedure used to create a vaginal canal is not important but that emphasis has to be placed on good preoperative psychosocial adjustment and good postoperative counselling and follow-up[4]. By evaluating each case on an individual basis and by choosing a less traumatic procedure like Vecchietti's operation the gynaecologist will be able to help the patient to adjust to her vaginal anomaly and to lead a full sexual life.

References

1. Frank, R.T. (1938). The formation of an artificial vagina without operation. *Am. J. Obstet. Gynecol.*, **35**, 1053
2. Vecchietti, G. and Ardillo, L. (1970). *La Sindrome de Rockitansky-Küster-Hauser. Fisiopatologia e Clinica.* (Rome: Societá Editrice Universo)
3. Vecchietti, G. (1980). Die Neovagina beim Rockitansky-Küster-Hauser Syndrom. *Gynäkologe*, **13**, 112
4. Hecker, B.R. and MacGuire, L.S. (1977). Psychosocial function in women treated for vaginal agenesis. *Am. J. Obstet. Gynecol.*, **129**, 543

53
Canalization of mucus in human fertility

S. CAMPO, E. GIACCHI, M. MESSINA, V. PANETTA
and N. GARCEA

INTRODUCTION

The importance of cervical mucus in the physiopathology of reproduction is considerable. It is the first barrier encountered by the spermatozoa on their route towards the ovum. The mechanisms which render the mucus permeable to the spermatozoa are still not clear; they probably depend upon variations in the number and quality of chemical bindings between the proteic macromolecules that constitute the structure of the mucus under the influence of the ovarian steroids.

Using Nuclear Magnetic Resonance techniques, Odeblad[1] has suggested that in the periovulatory phase the glycoproteic macromolecules form a linear pattern, while in the luteal phase the chains form a dense and compact grid. These structrual hypotheses have been confirmed with electronic microscope[2] and laser light-scattering spectroscopy[3].

In 1946 Papanicolaou[4] described the crystallization into fern leaves of cervical mucus. In 1971 Davajan[5] was the first to demonstrate the formation of 'channels' between the dendritic crystals of cervical mucus dried on a slide covered by a coverslip and examined through a microscope.

The aim of our study was:

(1) To study the canalization of cervical mucus in spontaneous ovulatory cycles,
(2) To study the biochemical bases of the phenomenon,
(3) To verify the oestrogen-dependence of canalization,

(4) To examine the action of drugs used for the inducement of ovulation (anti-oestrogens and gonadotropins) on canalization, and
(5) To correlate ferning and canalization, in order to demonstrate the greater reliability of canalization compared to ferning for the prediction of ovulation.

MATERIALS AND METHODS

We studied canalization in:

(1) 6 patients with spontaneous ovulatory cycles,
(2) 5 patients with primary amenorrhoea treated with ethinyl-oestradiol 0.02 mg/die and oestradiol-17β-valerate 2 mg/die for 6 days,
(3) 13 patients under treatment for the inducement of ovulation with HMG+HCG, and
(4) 7 patients treated with anti-oestrogens (5 with clomiphene 50 mg/die for 5 days and 2 with tamoxiphene 20 mg/die for 5 days).

The cervical mucus was collected each day with a sterile pipette, after cleaning the portio, and smeared onto a slide which was half covered by a coverslip.

The samples were examined under a Zeiss optical microscope ($\times$120). Blood samples were also obtained each day in order to measure E_2 and P by RIA (kit from Serono, Italy), FSH and LH (kit by Biodata, Italy).

We further studied ferning and canalization on 6 samples of periovulatory mucus:

(1) Before and after dialysis with H_2O for 24 hours, and 6 and 24 hours after the addition of 0.9 mmol/l NaCl to the dialysate;
(2) Before and after treatment with 0.5% trypsin, 100 μl for 1 hour.

RESULTS AND DISCUSSION

The number and arrangement of the channels varies during the different phases of the menstrual cycle. In the proliferative phase the channels appear around the 7th day and increase progressively in number until a maximum is reached in the periovulatory phase. In this period they form a linear arrangement. In the luteal phase they gradually decrease in number and take on a disordered pattern.

Figure 1 shows corresponding aspects of the crystallization of cervical mucus into channels and into fern leaves, both in the periovulatory (top) and initial luteal (bottom) phases. In the former, the parallel pattern of the channels is evident; in the latter, the pattern is mainly reticular.

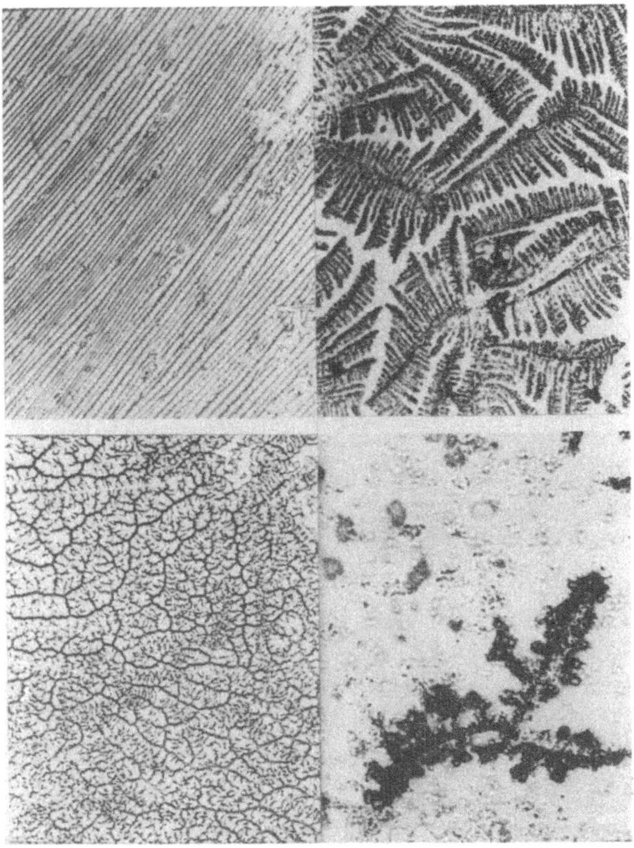

Figure 1 Ferning and canalization of the same sample of periovulatory cervical mucus (top) and luteal mucus (bottom)

The time required for canalization is 72 hours at room temperature[5,6]. We confirmed that *in vitro* canalization takes place in 6 hours at 40 °C and in 2 hours at 50 °C.

The presence of salts and proteins is essential for the phenomenon to take place. Dialysis of periovulatory mucus for 24 hours in fact caused ferning and canalization to disappear. The addition to the dialysate of a solution of 0.9 mmol/l NaCl caused initial crystallization to appear after 6 hours; after 24 hours typical ferning and typical canalization appeared.

Treatment with trypsin caused both ferning and canalization to disappear. Canalization is hormone-dependent.

In spontaneous ovulatory cycles the number of channels increases to reach a

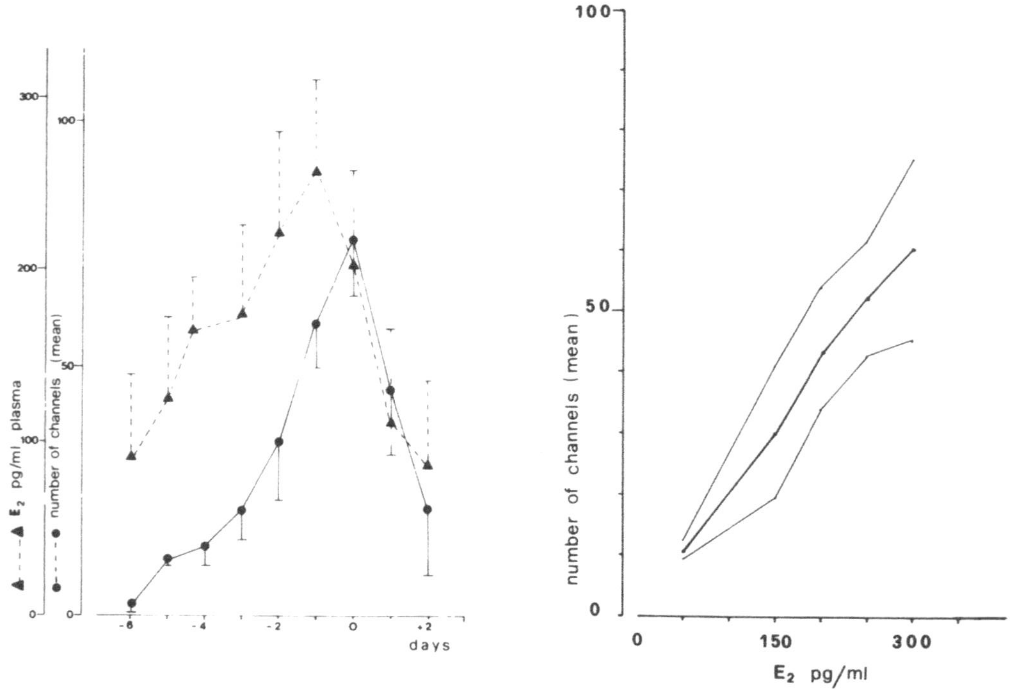

Figure 2 Correlation between the increase in channels and oestradiol (left). Day 'O' corresponds to the LH peak. (Right) relationship between E_2 levels and channels

maximum (75±11) at the same time as the LH peak. This increase parallels that of oestradiol, with a biological inertia time of 24 hours (Figure 2).

Treatment with oestrogens of five patients with primary amenorrhoea caused the appearance of canalization of the cervical mucus. Ethinyl-oestradiol was shown to be more effective than oestradiol-17β-valerate, probably acting directly on the receptors of the cervical glands (Figure 3).

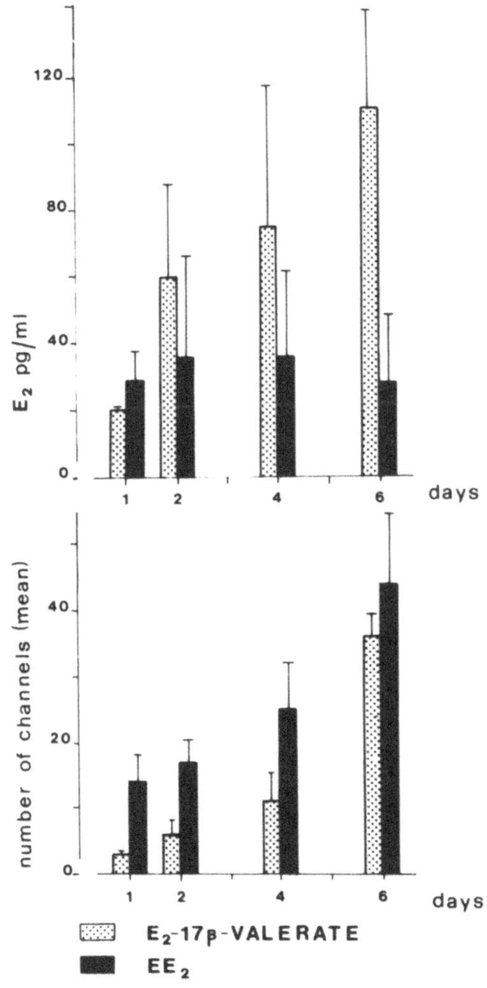

Figure 3 Effect of the administration of oestrogens on canalization in patients with primary amenorrhoea

The anti-oestrogens, clomiphene and tamoxiphene, have no negative effect on canalization.

In patients treated with anti-oestrogens the number of channels on the day of the LH peak was equal to that in the control patients, even in those patients in whom clomiphene had caused a reduction in the quantity of mucus. In these patients, too, we confirmed the parallel increase of oestradiol and channels with 24 hour inertia (Figure 4).

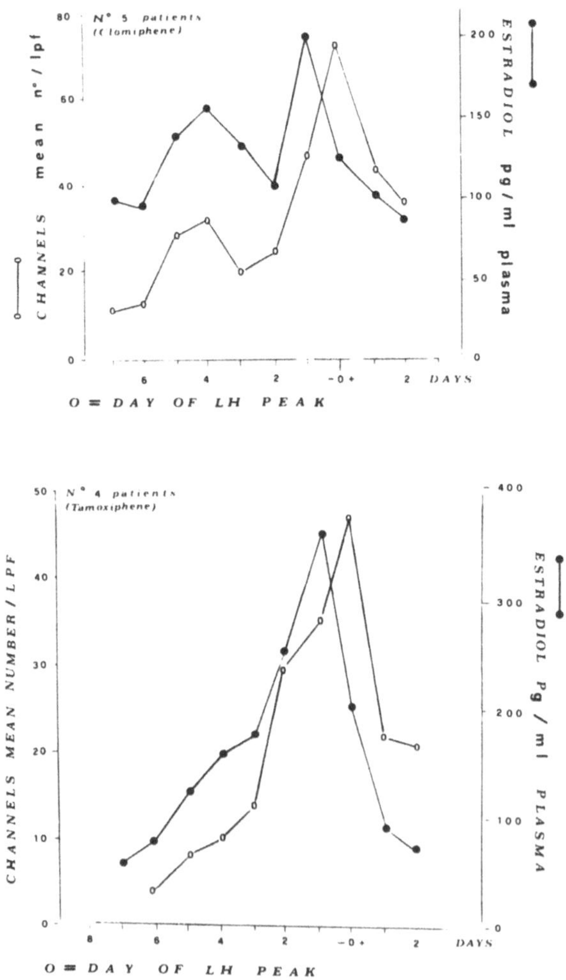

Figure 4 Relationship between E_2 levels and channels in patients treated with anti-oestrogens

Canalization is more reliable than ferning in monitoring ovulation.

An increase in the number of channels was also observed in patients stimulated with gonadotropins. It is interesting to emphasize that in 50% of women who did not conceive the number of channels on day 0 (day of HCG administration) was clearly lower than the average in those patients who did conceive, even though this difference is not statistically significant (Figure 5).

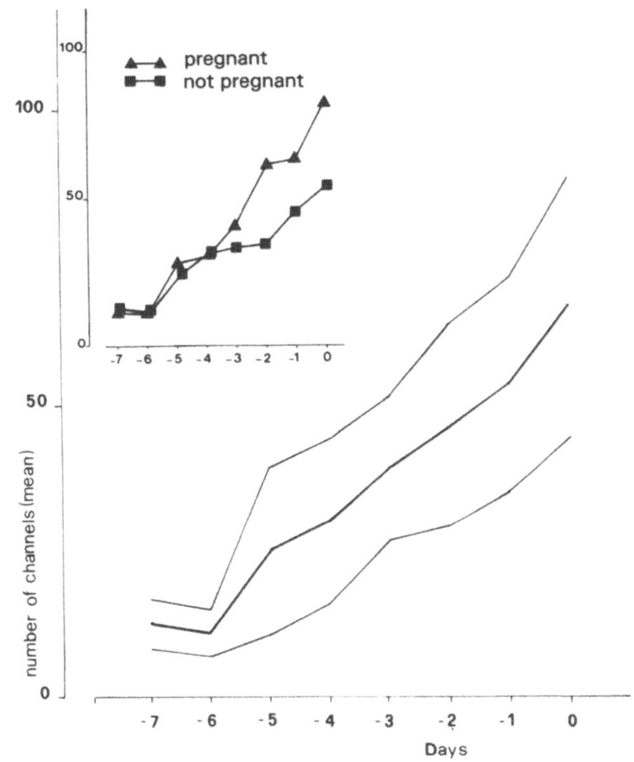

Figure 5 Increase in the number of channels during treatment with gonadotropins

The same grades of ferning[7] are observed on a number of consecutive days. On the other hand, the number of channels shows a progressive increase up to the LH peak. The 'static' phenomenon of ferning is thus set against a 'dynamic' phenomenon (canalization) as a parameter for oestrogenic activity (Figure 6).

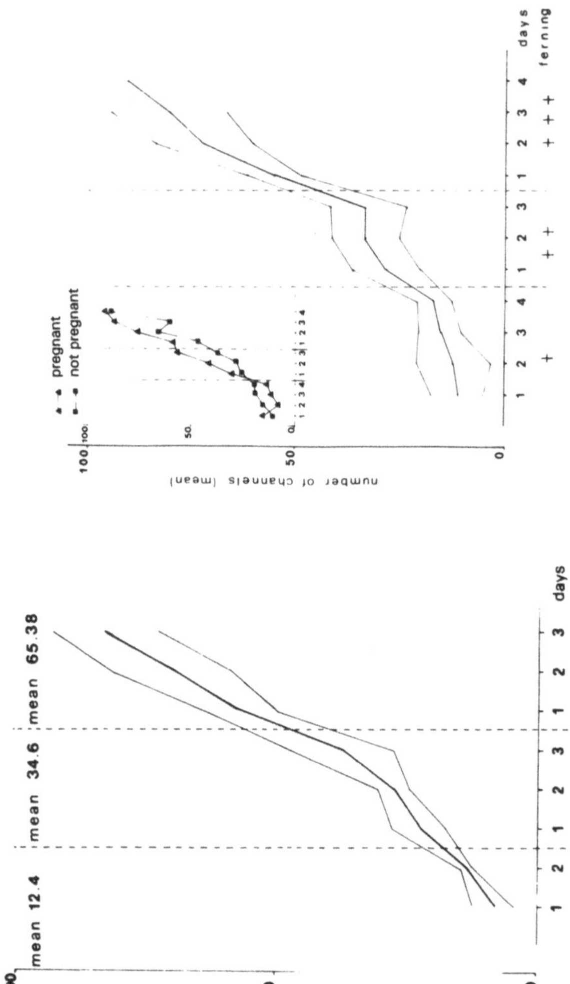

Figure 6 Relationship between grades of ferning and number of channels in spontaneous ovulatory cycles (left), and in ovulatory cycles induced with gonadotropins (right)

CONCLUSIONS

(1) The phenomenon of *in vitro* 'canalization' has the same biophysical characteristics as 'ferning'.

(2) Salts and proteins are essential for 'canalization' as they are for 'ferning'.

(3) The phenomenon is oestrogen-dependent.

(4) 'Ferning' requires subjective evaluation, while the 'number of channels' is quantifiable, and is therefore a more precise index of oestrogen levels and for the prediction of ovulation.

(5) The *in vitro* evidence of 'canalization' could be a demonstration of the hypothesis that the linear arrangement of the macromolecules of the mucus permits the spermatozoa to pass through the cervix during the ovulatory phase.

References

1. Odeblad, E. (1966). Micro-NMR in high permanent magnetic fields. Theoretical and experimental investigations with an application to the secretions from single glandular units in the human uterine cervix. *Acta Obstet, Gynecol. Scand.*, **45** (suppl. 2), 12
2. Chretien, F.C., Cohen, J. and Psychoyos, A. (1976). L'évolution de la trame ultra-structurale de la glaire cervicale humaine au cours du cycle ovarien. Etude au microscope électronique à balayage. *J. Gynécol. Obstét. Biol. Reprod.*, **5**, 313
3. Lee, W.J., Verdugo, P. and Blandau, R.J. (1977). Molecular arrangement of cervical mucus: a re-evaluation based on laser light-scattering spectroscopy. *Gynecol. Invest.*, **8**, 254
4. Papanicolaou, G.N. (1946). General survey of vaginal smear and its use in research and diagnosis. *Am. J. Obstet. Gynecol.*, **51**, 315
5. Davajan, V., Nakamura, R.M. and Mishell, D.R. (1971). A simplified technique for evaluation of the biophysical properties of cervical mucus. *Am. J. Obstet. Gynecol.*, **109**, 1042
6. Hilgers, T.W. and Prebil, A.M. (1979). The ovulation method. Vulvar observations as an index of fertility/infertility. *Obstet. Gynecol.*, **53**, 12
7. Roland, M. (1971). Can the fern test be graded? *Obstet. Gynecol.*, **37**, 782

54
Treatment of cervical mucus infection by means of doxycycline polyphosphate in 53 hypofertile women

J. BUVAT, M. BUVAT-HERBAUT, J. C. FOURLINNIE, F. DESMONS, C. CUVELIER, J. C. HERBAUT and A. LEMAIRE

INTRODUCTION

Cervical mucus infection is often considered as a possible cause of infertility[1]. Darugna *et al.* observed this abnormality in 13% of women consulting for infertility[2]. Nevertheless, pregnancies do occur in certain women whose cervical mucus is infected, and thus it is not an obligatory factor in proving sterility.

In order to study the effect of cervical mucus infection in infertility, we treated 53 infertile women whose cervical mucus was infected, by means of an antibiotic with a strong genital tropism: doxycycline polyphosphate (Doxycline-Laboratoires Plantier, France). Moreover, as *T.mycoplasma* (*Ureaplasma urealyticum*) and *Chlamydia trachomatis* are often implicated in infertility, we studied their role in cervical mucus infection by systematic investigations in our patients.

PATIENTS AND METHODS

Patients

Fifty-three women, infertile for more than 1 year, presented with a cervical mucus infection. This diagnosis was based on the presence of three criteria, observed at the time of the cervical mucus examination, during a preovulatory period or during oestrogenic treatment (100 μg ethinyl-oestradiol for 5–10 days):

(1) Alteration of the physical characteristics,
(2) Presence of numerous leukocytes,
(3) Presence of organisms in cervical mucus.

In order to interpret the pregnancy rate, the 53 patients were divided into three groups: Group A, 13 cases: no other known infertility factor in both partners. Group B, 26 cases: presence of one or two other infertility factors, theoretically treatable (dysovulation and/or oligoasthenospermia). Group C, 14 cases: presence of another infertility factor, untreatable (azoospermia or bilateral tubal stenosis).

Investigations

Each patient underwent the same investigations before and after treatment, each time in an identical hormonal context (preovulatory period or oestrogenic treatment). Cervical mucus was extracted in the laboratory by means of endocervical aspiration, after the exocervix was cleaned. Its physical properties (clarity, spinnbarkeit, ferning) and its leukocyte content were evaluated. Cervical mucus was cultured, in the usual culture media, for aerobic organisms. *Chlamydia trachomatis* and *Ureaplasma urealyticum* were cultured after endocervical scraping by means of a currette with a streaked extremity, then inoculation on MacCoy cells, and on a culture media for mycoplasma (kit IPP).

Treatment

Doxycycline polyphosphate was given for 6–8 weeks (saturation dose of 200 mg, then 100 mg twice a day, *per os*). No associated treatment was given to the other partner, except in certain cases in group B where treatment for infertility was begun more than 3 months before doxycycline treatment was started.

RESULTS

Bacteriological examinations of cervical mucus

Before treatment, 60 different organisms belonging to 8 different families were found in the 53 women (Table 1). *Ureaplasma urealyticum* was found six times, and *Chlamydia trachomatis* only once. After treatment, the initial infection had disappeared in 37 out of the 49 control women (75.5% of the cases). But in 18 out of these 37 cases a new organism was found (Table 1).

Table 1 Results of the bacteriological study of cervical mucus infection, before and after doxycycline polyphosphate treatment. In some cases two organisms were found in the same woman. Four cases could not be controlled because a pregnancy occurred before the end of treatment

		Cervical mucus		
	Before treatment	*After treatment*		
Organism		*Disappeared*	*Persistent*	*Appeared*
Chlamydia trachomatis	1	1	—	—
Ureaplasma urealyticum	6	6	—	—
Escherichia coli	20	14	5	4
Streptococcus enterococcus	18	10	6	11
Streptococcus group B	8	5	3	1
Staphylococcus aureus	4	4	—	—
Haemophilus vaginalis	2	2	—	—
Proteus mirabilis	1	1	—	2
Total	60	43	14	18

Cervical mucus: physical characteristics and cytology

After treatment, the physical characteristics were improved or normalized in 43% of the cases. Leukocytes were less numerous, or disappeared in 73.5% (Table 2).

Table 2 Effects of polyphosphate doxycycline treatment upon cervical mucus (CM) in 49 controlled cases

Physical properties	identical (28)	improved (12)	normalized (9)
Leukocytes	as numerous (13)	less numerous (15)	disappeared (21)
		Disappeared	
Initial organism	persistent (12)	+ a new germ (18)	sterile CM (19)

Pregnancies

Nine pregnancies occurred in the 4 months following the onset of antibiotic treatment (Group A, 4/13 women: (30%); Group B, 5/26 women: (19%).

COMMENTS

Chlamydia trachomatis and *Ureaplasma urealyticum* were only found in seven patients. In five of these cases, they were associated with another organism. So they rarely seem to be the cause of cervical mucus infections observed in infertile patients.

Doxycycline polyphosphate seems to have cured 75% of our cases of cervical mucus infection (disappearance of the initial organism and decrease or disappearance of leukocytes). The persistence of abnormalities of physical characteristics in certain cases could be explained by the after-effects of the infection at the level of the endocervical secretory epithelium. Nevertheless, the appearance of a new organism in 18 women is confusing. Although it is possible to find organisms in the healthy female endocervix[3], it is probable that, in certain cases, this new germ maintained the infection.

In Group A 30% of patients and in Group B 19% of patients became pregnant during the 4 months following the onset of the antibiotic treatment. Although our study has not included a control group, these numbers support the argument for a real role of cervical mucus infection in infertility in certain patients.

So, it seems logical to systematically treat cervical mucus infections in infertile women. First, this treatment can lead to pregnancies, but it also prevents the female upper genital tract and the partner from the risk of spread of the infection, that would constitute a source of new obstacles for fertility. Doxycycline polyphosphate seems to be an appropriate antibiotic for this systematic treatment. It has the advantage of being active against *Chlamydia trachomatis and Ureaplasma urealyticum*, the association of which with ordinary germs is possible, but, a not very well known fact is that they can endanger fertility without the association with other organisms.

References

1. Lansac, J., Laumosnet, J., Prieur, D. and Galtier, J. L. (1977). Infections de la glaire cervicale et fertilité. In *Infection et Fertilité*, p. 189. (Paris: Masson)
2. Darugna, D., Wenner, R. and Elö, Z. (1964). Le rôle de la cervicite et de la vaginite dans la stérilité. Les fonctions du col utérin. In *Colloque de la Société Nationale pour l'Etude de la Sterilité et de la Fécondité*, pp. 317–326. (Paris: Masson)
3. Moberg, P. J., Eneroth, P., Ljung, A. and Nord, C. E. (1979). Bacterial growth in samples from cervix and semen from infertile couples. *Int. J. Fertil.*, **24**, 157

Index

GPSR Compliance

The European Union's (EU) General Product Safety Regulation (GPSR) is a set of rules that requires consumer products to be safe and our obligations to ensure this.

If you have any concerns about our products, you can contact us on ProductSafety@springernature.com

In case Publisher is established outside the EU, the EU authorized representative is:

Springer Nature Customer Service Center GmbH
Europaplatz 3
69115 Heidelberg, Germany

Batch number: 10607222

Printed by Printforce, the Netherlands